THE MAUDSLEY
Maudsley Monographs

MAUDSLEY MONOGRAPHS

HENRY MAUDSLEY, from whom the series of monographs takes its name, was the founder of The Maudsley Hospital and the most prominent English psychiatrist of his generation. The Maudsley Hospital was united with the Bethlem Royal Hospital in 1948 and its medical school, renamed the Institute of Psychiatry at the same time, became a constituent part of the British Postgraduate Medical Federation. It is now associated with King's College, London, and entrusted with the duty of advancing psychiatry by teaching and research. The Bethlem-Maudsley NHS Trust, together with the Institute of Psychiatry, are jointly known as The Maudsley.

The monograph series reports work carried out at The Maudsley. Some of the monographs are directly concerned with clinical problems; others, less obviously relevant, are in scientific fields that are cultivated for the furtherance of psychiatry.

Maudsley Monographs number forty-two

Mental Health in our Future Cities

edited by

David Goldberg
and
Graham Thornicroft
Institute of Psychiatry, London, UK

Psychology Press
Taylor & Francis Group
HOVE AND NEW YORK

First published 1998 by Psychology Press
27 Church Road, Hove, East Sussex BN3 2FA

Simultaneously published in the USA and Canada
by Psychology Press
711 Third Avenue, New York, NY 10017

First issued in paperback 2014

Psychology Press is an imprint of the Taylor and Francis Group, an informa business

British Library Cataloguing in Publication Data

A catalogue record for this book is available from the British Library

ISSN 0076–5465

Cover design by Joyce Chester

Publisher's Note
The publisher has gone to great lengths to ensure the quality of this reprint but points out that some imperfections in the original may be apparent.

ISBN 13: 978-1-138-88449-6 (pbk)
ISBN 13: 978-0-86377-546-8 (hbk)

Contents

List of contributors

Deborah Agus, JD, 2200 Arden Road, Baltimore, MD 21209, USA.

Francesco Amaddeo, Istituto di Psichiatria, Università di Verona, Ospedale Policlinico, Via delle Menegone, 37134 Verona, Italy.

Gavin Andrews, Clinical Research Unit for Anxiety Disorders, University of New South Wales, 299 Forbes Street, Dalinghurst, NSW 2010, Australia.

Dinarte A.P. Ballester, Fundação Faculdade Federal de Ciências Médicas de Porto Alegre, Departamento de Psiquiatria e Medicina Legal, Rua Sarmento Leite, 245, 90050–170 Porto Alegre, RS Brazil.

Stephen T. Baron, President, Baltimore Mental Health Systems Inc, 201 E. Baltimore Street, Suite 1340, Baltimore, MD 21202, USA.

David Brown, Baltimore Crisis Response Inc., 1105 Light Street, 2nd Floor, Baltimore, MD 21201, USA.

Lorenzo Burti, Istituto di Psichiatria, Università di Verona, Ospedale Policlinico, Via delle Mnegone, 37134 Verona, Italy.

Ellis D'Arrigo Busnello, Fundação Faculdade Federal de Ciências Médicas de Porto Alegre, Departamento de Psiquiatria e Medicina Legal, Rua Sarmento Leite, 245, 90050–170 Porto Alegre, RS Brazil.

Miriam Dias, Secretaria Municipal de Saúde, Av. João Pessoa, 325, 90040–000, Porto Alegre, RS Brazil.

Maria de Fátima Fischer, Secretaria Municipal de Saúde, Av. João Pessoa, 325, 90040–000, Porto Alegre, RS Brazil.

Nicola Garzotto, Istituto di Psichiatria, Università di Verona, Ospedale Policlinico, Via delle Menegone, 37134 Verona, Italy.

Ariadne Runte Geidel, Escola Especial Municipal Luis Francisco Lucena Borges, Rua Cláudio Manoel da Costa, 270, 90000–000, Porto Alegre, RS Brazil.

Ad L.J. Goethals, APCP, Quellijnstraat 89, 1072 ZA Amsterdam, The Netherlands.

David Goldberg, Professor of Psychiatry, Institute of Psychiatry, De Crespigny Park, London SE5 8AF, UK.

Eric Hoffmann, APCP, Quellijnstraat 89, 1072 ZA Amsterdam, The Netherlands.

Cathy Issakidis, Clinical Research Unit for Anxiety Disorders, University of New South Wales, 299 Forbes Street, Darlinghurst, NSW 2010, Australia.

Marianne Kastrup, Department of Psychiatry, Copenhagen University Hospital, Hvidovre, 2650 Hvidovre, Denmark.

Mariko Kimura, Associate Professor in Social Work, Section of Social Welfare, Department of Health Services, Tokai University, Bousei-Dai, Isehara City, Kanagawa Prefecture, 259–11, Japan.

David LeCount, Dane County Department of Human Services, 1202 Northport Drive, Madison, Wisconsin 53704, USA.

Ahmad Mohit, Associate Professor and Former Chairman, Department of Psychiatry, Iran University of Medical Sciences, (Tehran Psychiatric Institute), Tehran, Iran.

R. Srinivasa Murthy, Professor of Psychiatry, Department of Psychiatry, National Institute of Mental Health and Neuro Sciences, Post Bag 2900 Bangalore 560 029, India.

Fred Osher, Associate Professor, Director, Division of Community Psychiatry, University of Maryland School of Medicine, 701 W. Pratt Street, 3rd Floor, Baltimore, MD 21201, USA.

Mirella Ruggeri, Istituto di Psichiatria, Università di Verona, Ospedale Policlinico, Via delle Menegone, 37134 Verona, Italy.

Norman Sartorius, Department de Psychiatrie, Hôpitaux Universitaires de Genève, 16–18 Boulevard de St Georges, 1205 Geneva, Switzerland.

Aart H. Schene, Academic Medical Centre, University of Amsterdam, P.O. Box 22700, 1100 DE Amsterdam, The Netherlands.

Naotake Shinfuku, Professor in International Health and Epidemiology, International Center for Medical Research, Kobe University School of Medicine, Kusunoki-cho, 7 chome, Chuo-ku, Kobe, Japan 650–0017.

Susumu Sugawara, Yadokari-no-sato, Nakagawa 562, Oomiya-city, Saitama Prefecture, 330, Japan.

Michele Tansella, Istituto di Psichiatria, Università di Verona, Ospedale Policlinico, Via delle Menegone, 37134 Verona, Italy.

Graham Thornicroft, Professor of Community Psychiatry, Institute of Psychiatry, De Crespigny Park, London, SE5 8AF, UK.
Ana Cristina Tietzmann, Fundação Faculdade Federal de Ciências Médicas de Porto Alegre, Departamento de Psiquiatria e Medicina Legal, Rua Sarmento Leite, 245, 90050–170 Porto Alegre, RS Brazil.
Teruo Yanaka, Executive Director, Yadokari-no-sato, Nakagawa 562, Oomiya-city, Saitama Prefecture, 330, Japan.
Patricia Zillmer, Escola Especial Municipal Luis Francisco Lucena Borges, Rua Cláudio Manoel da Costa, 270, 90000–000, Porto Alegre, RS Brazil.

Introduction: Mental health in our future cities

This book presents some of the best of the ideas and practices in modern mental health services from around the world. It indicates directions that have been travelled, and describes arrangements that work in practice. It shows that partnerships between individuals, and between organisations, can achieve results that can inspire people, both where they occur and far away.

Across the world, cities are becoming larger, as populations drift from the country in urban areas. At the same time, the mentally ill are leaving the mental hospital, and new forms of care are being found in the community. The best ways in which services for the mentally ill can be organised in the community are still a matter for debate, and as cities become larger problems may become greater.

In 1997, the Bethlem Royal Hospital celebrated its 750th birthday, and the King's Fund for London celebrated its centenary. Both organisations arranged a series of events to celebrate their achievements, but one such celebration was arranged jointly between them. This was an international conference held on 27–29 October at which 10 cities from around the world were invited to describe their mental health services, so that examples of good practice could be shared. The chapters that follow are the background briefing papers prepared by each city, up-dated by each set of authors in the light of what they saw and heard at the conference. In particular, they have included sections on how they see probable future developments in their cities.

The conference was to have a feature that made it unique among discussions of the shape of mental health services across the world: we wished to have intense participation by the users of the services themselves, as well as hearing both from carers and from voluntary organisations. To this end the King's Fund organised a series of meetings with user's organisations across London, and took into account their views about those aspects of the mental health services that deserved a critical airing. We made discounted tickets available to users, and succeeded in attracting over 130 London users to the conference, in addition to those from other international cities. We also invited experts in community mental health from outside our two organisations to share in the discussions with users. The 42 workshops that resulted from these meetings are described in Chapter 13.

The cities were chosen on a number of criteria. The three most important were: that there was an innovation in service delivery that was unusual in that part of the world and had attracted international attention; that we needed to achieve a good geographic spread across the world; and that the possible collaborator in each city had to reply to our letters, and be prepared to undertake the considerable amount of preparatory work involved. We lost several potential cities because of continued non-response, but all of those who replied to our letters carried out all the preparatory work. The first duty of the professional in each city was to identify an English speaking user who could accompany them to London and participate in the conference. Other work included contacting users' organisations in their city, and assisting them in making a videotape of services as seen from the users' perspective. They also had to prepare the reports that formed the briefing papers for the conference, and to prepare slides—some of which form the illustrations to this book.

The videotapes prepared by each city were brilliantly successful, and they are available on a videotape that accompanies this book[1]. The tapes give an impression of each service that cannot be obtained in any other way, and bring the text of the book to life in relation to real people.

Eric Byers	Julia Neuberger
Chief Executive	Chief Executive
Bethlem Maudsley NHS Trust	King's Fund

---

[1] Copies of this book and its accompanying videotape can be obtained from the King's Fund Bookshop, 11–13 Cavendish Square, London W1M 0AN; fax 0171 307 2801.

CHAPTER ONE

Nearly forgotten: The mental health needs of an urbanised planet

Norman Sartorius
Hôpitaux Universitaires de Genève, Switzerland

INTRODUCTION

It is an amazing fact that governments of the world, faced with rampant urbanisation, have not developed a strategy for the provision of health care in cities. In some 30 years four-fifths of the world population—in developed and developing countries, will be living in urban areas. This represents a steady growth for industrialised countries and a revolutionary change for most of the others. It is easy to predict that this change will bring new health problems or magnify those currently facing health care in an unprecedented manner: it is also probable that a well formulated plan of action to counter these problems might make it easier to deal with them.

These predictions have to be considered against the background of three arrays of facts. The first concerns the size of future cities: it is very unlikely that cities will cease to grow when they reach the size of today's largest towns; judging from tendencies already visible in some developing countries the cities of the future will grow to unprecedented sizes—to agglomerations of dwellings of 20 or 30 million people. Megalopolises are not only cities grown big: they are likely to be different creatures—in the same vein as adults are not big children although they continue to belong to the same biological species when they are children and when they grow up. This change—a revolution in Hegelian sense—means that most of the knowledge and administrative skills developed to manage cities will be only partially applicable to deal with life of a megalopolis; that health care organisation as well as other social services will have to examine systematically the applicability of their current strategies and ways of functioning if they are to be useful. This change of size also means that cities will no longer have a decorative town hall and a ceremonial mayor: a future megalopolis the size of a country or even a group of countries, will have the political processes and powers of a country the size of Ukraine, or of all of the Nordic European countries taken together.

The second array of facts concerns the locus of fastest growth. Urban growth is already much faster in the developing than in the industrialised countries. Life in Third world towns, with all its dangers and shortcomings, is still better than life in rural areas. Towns act as an irresistible magnet for the populations in the rural areas. Villagers in many countries become exhausted by their battle against corrupt administration, failing crops, the harsh environment and consequences of disasters rendered ever more costly in human life because of growing population density. Their vital forces get sapped up feeding guerrilla wars, by economic difficulties reflecting speculations at faraway stock exchanges, by expenses of pharaonic buildings, and by the continuing presence of (often preventable) communicable diseases. The apparent easy availability of all things in cities also exerts its influence, as do stories of successes and easy lives that some of the first migrants to cities have been able to lead.

Villagers do not migrate to towns any longer in small numbers and slowly: their move to cities is massive. They bring with them their culture and their habits, their manner of life often incompatible with functioning of large aggregations of humans sharing a restricted area. They are at first amazed by all that can be obtained, then despondent because all this wealth cannot be theirs; their search for a better life then takes different paths, from work for minimal wages (and without protection) to crime, violence, and prostitution. Health care for newcomers to towns is neither that appropriate for the villages from which they came nor that of towns in which they now live.

Third world cities are not only growing faster than their counterparts in industrialised countries: they also differ from them in many other ways. The population density in Cairo in 1995 was 375 inhabitants per hectare and in Calcutta 220: in comparison London had 40, New York 44, and Frankfurt 26 inhabitants per hectare. The number of children and adolescents in the developing country cities is much higher than in the developed countries, reflecting the difference in demographic structure between those two types of countries in general. There are other differences, often neglected, that matter a great deal in organising health care; the number of abandoned children and adolescents without family, for example, in some developing countries (e.g. in Latin America) is much higher than in the developed countries and continues to grow at a fast rate.

The third set of facts concerns the dramatic changes of the demographic composition and function of rural areas, the main donors of population to cities in many countries. Young and able-bodied people are often the first to leave home, with the resulting increase in proportion of the disabled, elderly and those too young to leave the rural areas. In some instances those who fail to succeed in towns or become disabled because of working conditions return to villages, further decreasing the capacity of the rural areas to function independently.

Villages near towns become dependent on them and on demands that towns make. Modern agricultural production reduces employment opportunities in rural areas, greatly increasing the numbers of the rural proletariat and of seasonal migrant agricultural populations now reaching vast numbers, for example in the Americas. The change of production style in rural areas further contributes to the reasons for leaving villages and migrating to towns, without any hope or wish to return to the rural area.

MENTAL DISORDERS IN TOWNS

The prevalence of mental disorders in cities differs from that in rural areas. In China, for example, schizophrenia seems to be more prevalent in cities and learning disability in villages (Cooper & Sartorius, 1997); in the UK, a 1995 survey showed that depressive disorders, generalised anxiety and phobias are higher in urban areas than in rural areas (Meltzer, Gill, Petticrew, & Hinds, 1995). There are more lonely chronic mentally ill people in cities than in villages. The homeless mentally ill in urban areas of industrialised countries are comparable to vagrant psychotics described in developing countries. It is uncertain, however, whether the mortality of these two groups is similar. It is also probable that mental disorders linked to early brain damage should be more prevalent in areas—urban slums or remote villages—in which access to health care and appropriate nutrition is difficult: unfortunately, these are also areas in which statistics (or results of studies) about morbidity from mental illness and mental impairment are less reliable, if available at all.

Drug and alcohol dependence have been described as urban mental health problems: there are, however, many areas in the Third world in which rural areas are just as strongly hit by drug dependence problems as the populations of towns (e.g. Pakistan, Thailand), and there is little doubt about the ravages that alcohol abuse and dependence creates in rural areas in many countries.

Studies of schizophrenia showed differences in course and outcome of mental disorders between developing and developed countries. Systematic comparisons of course and outcome of schizophrenia and other mental disorders in urban and rural areas of developing and developed countries are however lacking and it is unlikely that such data will become available in the immediate future. What is true for major mental disorders such as schizophrenia may also be true for other mental disorders and for neurological disorders. Differences in the prevalence of mental disorders in urban and rural areas have also been described: there is however little agreement about the reasons for this differences which may well, at least in part, be the result of variations in course and outcome of diseases.

While there is some information about differences in the prevalence of mental disorders in urban and rural areas data about the differences in the severity of the psychosocial problems of cities are by and large lacking. Loneliness, anomia, stress-related disorders (e.g. hypertension) as well as various forms of antisocial behaviour (e.g. violence) are seen as being typical of cities: it is difficult to know whether the situations that have been described in cities of industrialised countries also exist in developing countries and to what extent they are qualitatively different from them. Violence has been epidemically and then endemically present in certain countries, in both rural and urban areas (e.g. Mexico, Colombia) and it is difficult to declare violence in those countries as a typically urban problem.

It may be that in the future the differences in prevalence rates of mental and physical disorders in towns and villages will diminish. In developing countries today, for example, people suffering from a chronic disease will move to towns where help for their condition is available and then stay there, thus increasing the prevalence of certain chronic diseases. The increased density of families that contained a person suffering from a mental disorder around hospitals has been demonstrated in the past in the USA: similar phenomena are even more visible in the newly created settlements at the doorsteps of mental hospitals, for example in front of the Aro Mental Hospital in Abeokuta, Nigeria. With the development of communications, i.e. roads and cheaper transport between towns and surrounding areas, this type of migration of selected groups of population might decrease, thus diminishing differences between towns and rural areas.

A recent report (Harvard Working Group on New and Resurgent Diseases, 1995) provides a gloomy forecast of diseases of the future by pointing out that infectious diseases remain the leading cause of death in the world and that numerous diseases that were considered to be under control have made their way back to the top of the killing charts. Diphtheria has emerged as a major killer of adults in the countries of the Community of Independent States (in Russia alone the number of cases doubled between 1985 and 1992). Malaria and tuberculosis are creating major problems in many countries. Plague has made its way back in India and cholera has emerged in Latin America. Dengue fever, haemorrhagic fever, yellow fever as well as some diseases about which little was known (e.g. Lyme disease, hanta virus syndrome, toxic shock syndrome, AIDS and Ehrlichiosis) have appeared on the lists of priorities for public health authorities. Changes of ecosystems, water management, major development programmes, pollution, and over-harvesting of certain species (e.g. fish) as well as other excesses of socio-economic development combined with an increasing vulnerability of the human organism seem to make it certain that communicable diseases will continue to grow and create public health problems—the major difference probably being that they will no longer be restricted only to rural or only to urban areas but will hit both areas, and in them particularly the poor, with similar power.

OPPORTUNITIES FOR HEALTH CARE INTERVENTIONS IN CITIES

At present urban areas offer opportunities for health care interventions that would be difficult to find in villages. The population is easier to reach in health campaigns. Health care personnel are concentrated in towns and are likely to stay there. Slum dwellers, particularly in the developing countries are resourceful and can be motivated to participate in health care activities. Funding for health care is easier to find. In-service training for personnel of health and other social services is easier to organise. Quality assurance of health care facilities is less complex. Supplies of health care materials are easier to organise. Laboratories can function more efficiently. Politicians and other individuals of high public visibility can be shown health services in difficulty and be involved in improving them. Gaps between academia and practice can be diminished and training of different categories of health care personnel can be carried out in health facilities serving the majority of the population.

Many of these opportunities for improving or providing health care in towns are not utilised; it is however important to remember them in defining health strategies for cities and in calculating investments that might be necessary to put urban health care into operation.

POSSIBLE AREAS OF ACTION

A prerequisite for the formulation of a useful and usable strategy is agreement on the meaning of terms and concepts used in its formulation. In the instance of a strategy for health care in cities, the meaning of many of the concepts that have to be used changed in the past few years. There is no commonly accepted definition of a city, or of a village, township or town. Villages previously inhabited by farmers toiling the land nearby have become inhabited by middle class and richer people from towns who establish secondary residences in those villages now being described as romantic, charming, quaint and culturally traditional. Townships have forever lost their previous meaning and now remain synonymous with the aggregations of prefabricated and concentration camp like structures established during apartheid in Zimbabwe and South Africa. Cities in the developing world have grown rapidly and often have the appearance of a huge camp of migrants or refugees situated around a dilapidated nucleus of a previously established small or medium sized town housing the administrative centre of a province or a country, built over the past 100 years or so. The periphery of the settlement may contain the newest migrants to town; but there are vast differences in the manner in which these towns have grown and in which the population groups that make up the town have distributed the space occupied by the city. In some instances the original tribes or villages re-establish themselves in the new settlement; in other instances the social class structure prevails and the rich live with the rich, the poor with the poor. Developed country towns have also become different from what has been described by writers, sociologists and demographers in the past six or eight decades, during which much of the writing on the subject was done. Inner city slums have been turned into expensive property and house the chic and rich; and the huge buildings or groups of buildings housing several thousand people have not infrequently turned into citadels, better depicted by artists in films or novels, than by scientists who seem to write little about the structure and functioning of such conglomerates. Currently growing gaps between scientific disciplines do not help to learn more about these matters: geographers who produced excellent descriptions of new urban arrangements rarely write in a manner that is attractive to doctors; and even if they did, it is unlikely that public health decision makers or psychiatrists would be following this literature.

Even the concepts of a street or a park have different meanings from one setting to another. The streets in which house numbers go up to 10,000 or more represent different concepts from the street in most European towns which never had more than a couple of hundred house numbers and in which it was highly probable that everybody knew everybody else. Towns that came into existence at different points of time bear characteristics of that time that distinguish them architecturally and functionally from one another, to a degree that makes it necessary that they organise the lives of their citizens and their health care in radically different ways. While basic medical skills required to work in towns may be similar, demographic features of a town—e.g. the preponderance of elderly persons, or of children—and various other characteristics of the city will require special or more skills in one area than in another.

Terms used to describe towns are not the only which have changed their meaning: the same is true for other frequently used notions and concepts, for example that of the community. A community was earlier defined as a population subgroup occupying a defined geographic area and having links of mutual support: nowadays, the criterion of living in the same area is only rarely useful. Links of mutual support are still important but do not, any longer, exist primarily among neighbours. People inhabiting the same geographical area in modern towns often do not know each other and have little in common with the exception of their address; links of support are defined differently, by family ties, by the enterprise employing the bread-winner, by minority or language grouping. Administrative authorities still do not recognise this change of definition of community and establish community health centres, for example, that serve only a small subgroup of the population.

Nor is there agreement on the way in which the functioning of a town or the success of a health care intervention will be assessed. Indicators of change differ from one setting to another and their definition is often slightly but significantly different so that comparison across services, across towns or across time are flawed.

It would be too ambitious at present to seek acceptance of indicators of progress, on the definition of criteria, on methods of definition of areas of intervention (e.g. of 'communities'), or criteria for the assessment of levels of priority, although this would be highly desirable. An immediate objective at present should be to work on the definition of terms in a manner that will allow their clear comprehension and a rational interpretation of the results of studies or of monitoring service interventions.

Next, it will be necessary to admit that towns have their personalities and that there is no such thing as a strict doctrine that will be applied in each case. The best that can be expected is agreement on certain principles that can serve as the frame for health care activities. These principles will have to be formulated, proclaimed and then used in developing plans, in educating the general public and in creating new generations of health workers. The essence of most of these principles can already be stated: the challenge is to formulate them sufficiently clearly for all to understand and use.

One such principle is that health care in cities can not and should not be planned or executed by the health care sector alone. This principle of multi-sectoral involvement has also been put forward in the Alma Ata Declaration: over time, it has been implemented in a number of settings, often with reluctance and usually with reservations. Successful services developed already, and described in the chapters that follow, show how health and social services can collaborate; how the voluntary sector can be included in mental health services; and how users themselves can contribute to the overall service. The political backing for multi-sectoral collaboration should not be sought as an afterthought: rather it will be of importance to assert that no significant improvement of health in cities can be expected until and unless the political authorities and leaders make that their own priority and force the administrative authorities to find structures and manners of function that will ensure collaborative action that will result in better quality of life of citizens. Those that can demonstrate that their efforts can make a significant contribution to that goal can then be given an opportunity to do so.

It is also clear that long-term planning in conditions of rapid social change and amid economic upheavals can not be realistic. While general principles of health care—such as equity in distributing benefits of health care and parity in service provision for mental and physical disorders—must be stated and used as a framework for short-term specific plans, 'rolling horizon' planning and programming are imperative: in order to make them possible and realistic, resources of health care services will have to be structured in a manner that will allow changes in the direction of care or a major re-orientation of activity in a short time.

Parallel to the principle of flexibility must be the principle of accountability and transparency of expenditure and investment. If the population is to be a willing partner to health care authorities it must be given respect and opportunities to see what is going on and what its own contribution to health care might be. In the first instance this will involve a major investment in a different type of health education—education on how to plan, execute and evaluate health care programmes. Health education of the type that was promoted previously—for example on the reproductive cycle of disease vectors—will have to continue but should not be seen as sufficient for health care purposes.

The acceptance of the population as an equal partner in the planning and execution of health care requires a significant change of the definition of the health professions and their life course: this is however the price to pay if a new paradigm of health care is to be introduced. A corollary of these principles is that investments have also to be made in activities that will promote health and mental health on the scale of values of individuals and communities. Once the population values health highly it will be willing to participate in efforts to prevent diseases or make arrangements for their treatment (Sartorius, 1998).

Another principle that might be useful for the improvement of mental health care in cities is that progress should be achieved by learning from others—in the same country or elsewhere—and by sharing one's experience with them. This commonality in progress will involve the creation of networks of information exchange and the development of an attitude of humility about one's own achievements or country. This volume is an important step in that direction.

CODA AND INVITATION

Thirty years ago, the World Health Assembly that brings together Ministers of Health or their envoys from the member countries of the World Health Organization expressed appreciation and unanimously adopted the various measures that were necessary to put the Alma Ata Declaration on primary health care into operation. The Declaration and the documents that accompanied it defined a new strategy of health care for the world. It introduced principles and guidelines that directed health systems into a new manner of operation. It underlined the need for delegation of most of health care tasks to relatively simply trained personnel, the imperative necessity to rationalise health care expenditures, the unavoidable assignation of priorities to health problems, the need for new alliances between health and other social sectors in all health care action and the usefulness of monitoring progress and achievements. Primary health care was a strategy (Sartorius, 1997) expressing the manner in which health care should reflect ethical principles governing societies at the end of the 20th century. It harnessed energy, knowledge and good will of many into a common framework of health care for the next three decades.

Useful as it might have been at the time of its formulation, the Primary Health Care strategy was deficient in that its prescription was primarily applicable to developing countries and in them, to care in rural areas. It did not anticipate changes in the trends of urban development nor foresee a viable mechanism for its own evaluation and revision in time. It was clearly overawed by the magnitude of health problems of the 1970s and captured in the political tensions that prevailed at the time of its formulation.

The consequences of these shortcomings are emerging in a variety of ways. Primary health care as a single strategy and as the only locus of investment in the health care system has lost its appeal in many countries and for most of the public health and other decision makers. Faced with urban health problems and changes in the rural areas ministries of health and social welfare employ a variety of strategies that are often in part or in their totality contradictory to one another although concocted in the same country or even in the same city at two points of time. Health plans are based on obsolete public health notions and lack foresight. Investments into health care are spasmodic and often governed by the need to deal with yet another crisis. Data on which public health action should be based are not collected regularly, or are losing credibility for a variety of (usually political and managerial) reasons. Economic imperatives are invoked to justify decisions whose ethical features are often at the very limit of acceptability. The complex mental health systems, involving many agencies and bringing together expertise from different sources that are described in the pages that follow are examples of the sort of systems that will need to be developed. They go well beyond a simple reliance on primary care services as the remedy for all problems.

Mental health problems of cities of today and even more of tomorrow are many and severe. They complement and aggravate other health problems that endanger existence and quality of life of citizens of urban and rural areas. They must be faced and overcome if the majority of mankind is to have a future worth living.

The formulation of a strategy to overcome mental and other health problems of the cities of the future will have to proceed in an inductive manner, basing its formulation on examples of successes often achieved under conditions of tremendous scarcity and deprivation of resources of all types. It will have to draw its strength from the motivation and creative power that was demonstrated in towns that have developed mental health and other health services. It will have to use the experience gained in developing health care and in many other areas of humanitarian effort.

Developing strategies and services that can provide appropriate health care for the cities of tomorrow is a venture of survival in an unknown territory replete with problems but also with promises of progress in a material and moral sense. In this game success will depend more than ever before on the collaboration of many, on the creation of a productive alliance between the population at large, patients and users of health services, scientists, health professionals, decision makers in the fields of health, mental health and other industry, nationally and internationally.

The principles for action proposed above are a personal choice. Their enumeration will have achieved its purpose if the list will stimulate the formulation of a list of tenets for urban development—including the development of urban health and mental health care. Reaching agreement on these tenets, the creation of a strategy formulated jointly by all concerned and then used by them, is an essential task for all of us at the point of entry into a new millennium in which people should not only end up by being in cities but should share a determination of making cities a liveable place, in which they can grow together and continue to improve the quality of life for themselves and for all those who will follow them in time.

REFERENCES

Cooper, J.E., & Sartorius, N. (Eds) (1996) *Mental disorders in China. Results of the National Epidemiological Survey in 12 areas.* London: Gaskell.

Harvard Working Group on New and Resurgent Diseases (1995). New and resurgent diseases: The failure of attempted eradication. *The Ecologist, 25,* 21–26.

Meltzer, H., Gill, B., Petticrew, M., & Hinds, K. (1995) *The prevalence of psychiatric morbidity among adults living in private households.* London: HMSO.

Sartorius, N. (1997). Psychiatry in the framework of primary health care: A threat or boost to psychiatry. *American Journal of Psychiatry, 154*, Festschrift Suppl.
Sartorius, N. (1998). Universal strategies for the prevention of mental illness and the promotion of mental health. In: R. Jenkins & T.B. Üstün (Eds), *Preventing mental illness—mental health promotion in primary care.* Chichester: John Wiley & Sons.

CHAPTER TWO

London's mental health services

Graham Thornicroft and David Goldberg
Institute of Psychiatry, London, UK

London is one of the world's great cities, and with other large conurbations it shares a mix of concentrated urban social diversity that both produces the high levels of demand for mental health services, and requires a subtlety of response commensurate with the needs of its populations. In this chapter we shall give an overview of the national context of mental health services in the UK, describe the particular socio-demographic features of London which are important to understand mental health needs, and summarise the results of a recent study which is the most detailed account yet undertaken of the conditions and the adequacy of the services providing psychiatric treatment and support in the capital (Johnson, Ramsay, Thornicroft, Brooks, & Lelliot et al., 1997). We paint a picture which is a mosaic composed of fragments of excellence, surrounded by a background tone of a service stretched to its maximum capacity. In the final chapter of this book we shall compare London's services with those featured in the other chapters, in terms of resources, performance and quality.

London has a population of almost 7 million people, representing approximately 14% of the population of England and Wales. The Boroughs range in size from 138,000 in Kingston upon Thames to 305,000 in Barnet. In this chapter the term 'London' is used to describe the 32 Boroughs which correspond to the area of the former Greater London Council (1936–86). The GLC covered an area defined by 1938 legislation on the metropolitan green belt—this was based on the extent of contiguous urban development at that time. Sixteen health purchasing authorities now cover an area almost co-terminous with that occupied by these London Boroughs. Within this area, acute mental health services were delivered, until recently, by 27 National Health Service (NHS) Trusts (service provider units).

CONTEXT OF MENTAL HEALTH SERVICES IN THE UK

In-patient care

From a peak in 1954 of 152,000, the number of people occupying psychiatric beds fell by 74% to 39,500 in 1993 (HMSO, 1994). The location of psychiatric beds has also changed. As the large, single-speciality hospitals were run down, beds were placed increasingly in small units, often in district general hospitals. This process was in its early stages in 1985. By March 1993 there were still about 20,500 patients in large hospitals, 52% of the national total patient population. Thirty-eight of the original 130 'water tower hospitals' had actually closed at this date (Davidge, Elias, Jayes, Wood, & Yates, 1993). The proportion of patients in large psychiatric hospital beds who were under 65 years (52%) resembles closely the proportion for all NHS psychiatric beds. This, together with the fairly low average length of stay (76 days) suggests that the beds in large hospitals were used for similar purposes to those in other settings. Figure 2.1 shows the declining overall numbers of residents in hospitals over this period.

Between 1969 and 1991, a period which saw the number of hospital residents fall by two-thirds, the number of admissions per 100,000 pop-

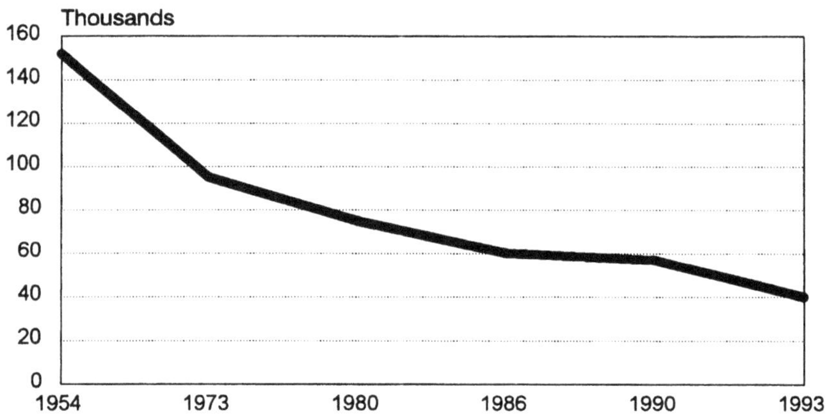

FIG. 2.1. Residents in hospital psychiatric in-patient units.

ulation actually increased by 8% (from 371 to 399 per 100,000). This was possible largely because of a great reduction in the number of resident patients with protracted lengths of stay. In 1991, 65% of discharged patients had lengths of stay of less than one month, and 90% less than three years. After remaining constant since the Mental Health Act was amended in 1983, the absolute number of compulsory admissions increased by 27% between 1989 and 1993, although this only represents an increase from 7.4% to 8.1% of all admissions.

Non-hospital residential provision

Not all NHS hospital beds which have been closed have been replaced by residential places provided by other agencies and in other settings. Over the last decade for which there are complete data (1983–1993), 29,330 NHS psychiatric beds closed, a 43% reduction in provision, and 7700 new places opened in residential facilities managed by other agencies. This represents replacement of only 26% of the beds lost (HMSO, 1994). More than 80% of these new residential places were provided by the voluntary and private sector, the remainder by local authorities.

This changing pattern of provision has meant that by 1993, 27% of residential provision was managed by agencies other than the NHS, compared with just 9% in 1983. As the balance of provider agency has shifted so has the nature of the residential provision available to the mentally ill. While almost all psychiatric hospital beds have 24-hour cover with nursing staff on duty and awake at night, residential accommodation provided by other agencies is much less likely to have such high staffing levels.

Day hospitals and day centres

Figure 2.2 shows changes in the total numbers of places in day hospitals and day centres over the last 15 years. Following a 73% increase during the 1980s, from 12,950 in 1979 to 22,400 in 1989, the number of psychiatric day hospital places has remained virtually static since with 22,900 in 1993 (HMSO, 1994). During this recent period the number of total attendances was unchanged but the number of new attendances increased by 13% (from 56,000 in 1989 to 72,000 in 1994) (Department of Health, 1998). Day centre places provided by local authorities for mentally ill people under 65 years increased by 74% (from 8700 to 15,100) during the decade up to 1992 (HMSO, 1994).

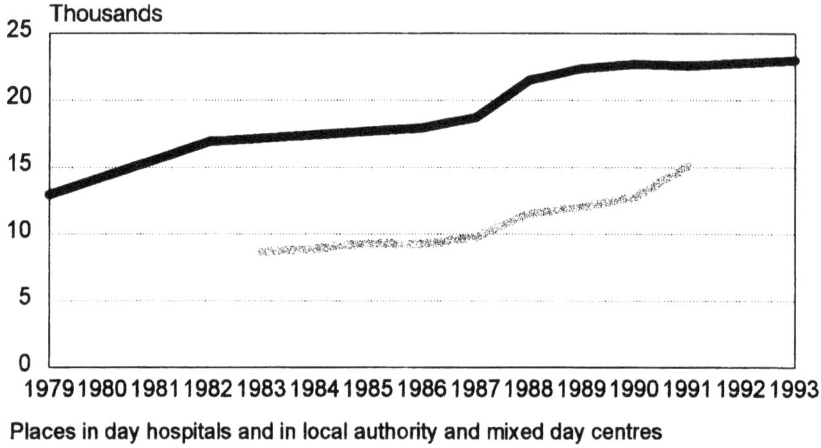

FIG. 2.2. Trends in day care provision. ▬, day hospital; ░, day centres.

LEVELS OF MENTAL HEALTH SERVICE NEED IN LONDON

The evidence supporting the view that Londoners' mental health needs are at the extreme end of the spectrum comes from two major sources. First, there are a number of socio-demographic indicator variables which have been found to have marked influences on the prevalence of psychiatric disorders and on mental health service utilisation. These characteristics include rates of unemployment and homelessness, ethnic composition of the population, age structure, and overall social deprivation. This chapter will begin by describing those socio-demographic characteristics of London which are likely to have a significant impact on its population's needs for mental health services. We shall focus here upon three of the most relevant issues: social deprivation, age structure and ethnic minority groups, although other factors such as homelessness, household composition, residential mobility and unemployment will also tend to raise the level of demand for mental health services in the capital.

Social deprivation

The relationship between psychiatric disorder and various measures of poverty, low social class or social deprivation began to be a major focus for research in psychiatric epidemiology early in the 20th century. Many positive findings have been reported since the original observation in the 1930s in Chicago that there was a higher rate of admission for psychosis in poorer central areas than in more prosperous outer areas. A series of subsequent studies have confirmed this tendency for people with psychotic disorders to be concentrated in inner cities.

More recently, exploration of the characteristics of areas which predict high rates of mental disorder has been aided by the development of specific indicators of social deprivation. In studying links between deprivation and psychiatric disorder at an area level, the most widely used composite indicator in recent UK research has been the Jarman index, or Under-Privileged Area score (UPA score), originally developed on the basis of general practitioners' observations about the characteristics of populations which had the most marked effects on their workloads. Use will be made of this indicator in later parts of this chapter. It has been shown to be highly correlated with psychiatric admission rates for health districts in London (Thornicroft, 1991) and across the whole of England (Jarman, Hirsch, White, & Driscoll, 1992).

The UK National Morbidity Survey, a large community survey, has recently indicated that the highest overall rates of neurotic disorders and of drug and alcohol dependence are in social classes IV and V (Meltzer, Gill, Petticrew, & Hinds, 1995). In fact, the extent of deprivation in inner London may be increasing. Between the censuses of 1981 and 1991, proxy indicators for poverty and wealth from the census (unemployment, economic inactivity, socio-economic group, car ownership and educational attainment), show evidence of relative increases in the degree, extent and intensity of poverty in inner London. Thus population-level composite indicators of deprivation already suggest that Londoners' mental health needs may be particularly great.

Age structure

London deviates markedly from the rest of the country in its age structure, in that the city as a whole and the inner city in particular has proportionately more young people than England and Wales as a whole. OPCS mid-year estimates for the year 1993 showed that in inner London, 36.3% of the population was aged between 15 and 45 compared with 29.4% in England and Wales (OPCS, 1993). London has a lower proportion of elderly people than England and Wales as a whole, and again this is particularly marked for inner London, where 12.6% were over 65 in 1993, compared with 15.9% nationally. There is often a pattern of young people from other parts of the country initially moving into central London, but later, as they get older, moving to outer London suburbs and beyond.

This difference in age structure has significance for population needs for mental health services. Most people with psychotic illnesses present to services for the first time below the age of 45, and research on the course of psychotic illness suggests that for the majority, needs for admission and social care will be greatest during the earlier years of the illness. Eating disorders, drug abuse and personality disorders are other forms of psychiatric disorder for which epidemiological evidence suggests that young adults are likely to have the greatest needs for services.

Ethnic minorities

Ethnic composition is another aspect of London in which it differs markedly from the remainder of the UK, even the other metropolitan areas. At the 1991 census, 45% of Britain's ethnic minority population was resident in London, and 20.3% of London's population was from an ethnic minority; 21.7% of London's population were born outside the UK, representing 38.4% of all such people resident in the country. The degree of concentration in London varies from community to community. Ethnic groups predominantly living in London rather than elsewhere in the country include Black Africans, with 77% of UK Black Africans resident in London, as well as 58% of the nation's population of Black Caribbeans and 52% of Bangladeshis. Almost all other major British minority communities apart from the Pakistani community are substantially over-represented in London.

The results of a number of studies have suggested that different communities have different patterns of prevalence of mental illness. The commonest focus in work of this type has been on the prevalence of psychosis among Black Caribbean people. Over the past decade, several studies, including some carried out in London, have indicated that Caribbean people are at higher risk than their White neighbours of being admitted to psychiatric hospital, or of being diagnosed as suffering from schizophrenia (King et al., 1994). The reasons for this repeated finding are uncertain, and it remains possible that it results more from the very high levels of social disadvantage experienced by this group than from any true ethnic difference.

Moreover, there is evidence that as well as possibly having different patterns of illness, mentally ill members of some minority ethnic communities have different patterns of service contact and report different experiences of the mental health services from the white community. Again the experiences of those members of the Black Caribbean community diagnosed as having psychotic illnesses have tended to dominate the debate. Overall, they appear less likely to have voluntary contact with the services and more likely to be subject to various forms of coercive control. Davies et al. (1996) have found much higher increased rates of detention under the Mental Health Act among both Africans and Afro-Caribbeans in a south London catchment area. In general there appears, at least among some sections of this community and its leaders, to be a strong feeling of alienation from the statutory services and of suspicion of these services. This sense that the services are failing many Black patients resonates with the conclusion of a series of reports and inquiries that services appear to have limited success in engaging this population in voluntary treatment.

Thus the remarkable ethnic diversity of Londoners is likely to lead to an increased requirement for resources and training to make services appropriate, and may also lead to a higher prevalence of psychiatric disorder. London is particularly distinctive in that, whilst other parts of the country have high concentrations of one or two ethnic groups, many areas of London are home to substantial numbers of members of a wide variety of different communities. Thus setting up parallel services for one or two ethnic groups will not usually meet local need comprehensively, and the ethnic sensitivity of generic services becomes a central issue.

THE KING'S FUND LONDON COMMISSION REPORT: 'LONDON'S MENTAL HEALTH'

In 1997 the King's Fund, an independent health service research and development agency, published the most detailed account yet undertaken of London's mental health services. The report was produced by a consortium of four research teams: the Section of Community Psychiatry (PRiSM) and Centre for the Economics of Mental Health (CEMH), both at the Institute of Psychiatry; the Centre for Mental Health Services Development (CMHSD), King's College London; and the Royal College of Psychiatrists Research Unit (CRU), reported in Johnson et al. (1997).

The questions addressed in the report included the following. Are the mental health needs of Londoners different in extent or degree from those of the rest of the UK's population? Does the functioning of London's mental health services differ from services in the rest of the country? How far has a community-based model of care been implemented in the city? What is the current evidence on the state of acute wards in London and on the availability of alternatives to admission? To what extent is a comprehensive range of facilities readily available for the city's mentally ill, including accommodation with a variety of levels of support, day care and leisure facilities, home support, advocacy services and employment schemes? Is there equity in London's provision, with the populations of different parts of the city and members of the many different ethnic minority communities all having their needs met to an equal extent? What costs are associated with current provision and what would be the resource implications for different areas of London of adopting innovative models of care? How might the capital's mental health services be improved so that they meet the mental health needs of Londoners more fully?

Provision in London compared with the rest of the UK

The Department of Health statistical division have data from the year 1994/5, which allows comparison between current service activity in London and that in the rest of the country. Figure 2.3 shows total number of psychiatric admission episodes, or Finished Consultant Episodes (FCEs) per 100,000 population for each geographical group, and rates for men and for women are shown separately.

Thus overall, inner London had the highest rate of admission episodes per 100,000 population of any of the four geographical groups and outer London the lowest. For all ages, inner London had 58% more FCEs per 100,000 than outer London, 9% more than other large cities and 37% more than the rest of the country. These differences were more marked for FCEs of people aged 16–64, where inner London has 83% more FCEs than outer London, 22% more than other large cities and 72% more than the rest of the country. Looking at data for men aged 16–64 only, the differences are still more pronounced, with inner London having a rate 94% above that of outer London, 33% above that of other large cities and 99% above the rest of the country (Johnson & Lelliot, 1997).

Levels of available in-patient and residential care services

To compare actual provision and estimated need and any gaps, we first conducted a detailed postal and telephone survey of provision throughout London. Details of the categories used are shown in Fig 2.4.

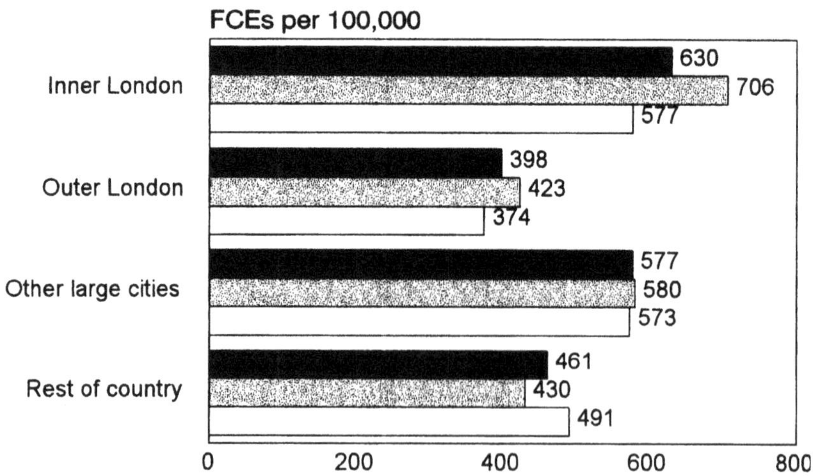

FIG. 2.3. Finished Consultant Episodes per 100,000—all ages. ■, all; ▩, men; □, women.
Source: Johnson et al., 1997

1. Regional secure beds
Medium secure beds in a regional secure unit.

2. Local secure beds
Low secure beds, for example, on an intensive care unit (ICU), special care unit or locked ward.

3. Acute beds
Acute beds or crisis beds for adults with serious mental illness requiring short-term admission to hospital, or occasionally, in the community.

4. Respite beds
Short-term beds for adults with chronic illness in hospital or community facilities.

5. Continuing care beds and hostel ward beds
Beds for adults with serious mental illness needing 24-hour care long-term, on or very close to, hospital estate.

6. 24-hours staffed Residential places
A high staffed hostel or residential home has awake or sleeping-in staff at night. Staff may be qualified or not qualified.

7. Lower support accommodation

7a. Day staffed residential places
A day staffed hostel or residential home has staff attending regularly for fixed hours, 4–7 days a week.

7b. Unstaffed hostel/group home places
Minimally supported hostels or residential homes with visiting staff. Include in this category any supported, self-contained flats with one or several staff on call in separate accommodation.

FIG. 2.4. Classification of types of in-patient and residential care

Estimated needs for such types of service were calculated using the given assumed service provision, full details of which are given by Johnson et al. (1997), based upon the Mental Illness Needs Index (Glover, 1996), as shown in Table 2.1.

TABLE 2.1
Estimated Need for General Adult Mental Health Services (aged 15–64 only), In-Patient and Residential Care, per 250,000 Population

Type of Service	*PRiSM Estimates of Need 1996*	*Actual Level of Provision*		
	Range	*Average Outer London*	*Average Inner London*	*Range in London*
1. Medium Secure Unit	5–30	8	26	0–58
2. Intensive Care Unit/ local secure unit	5–20	8	16	0–40
3. Acute ward	5–175	72	110	32–165
4. 24-hour nurse staffed units/ hostel wards/staff awake at night	12–50	50	38	0–158
5. 24-hour non-nurse staffed hostels/ night staff sleep-in	50–300	104	175	29–287
6. Day staffed hostels	15–60	17	50	17–292 for these two categories
7. Lower support accommodation	30–120	43	115	

How does expenditure compare with predicted need?

The Mental Illness Needs Index (MINI) has been widely used in the UK to predict the likely levels of facilities required in an area, when census tract data are taken into account (Glover, 1996). This is embodied in a computer program, which decides where in a range of published estimates for particular facilities a particular geographical area falls. We allowed the upper limits to reflect actual provision, and also made a number of other assumptions. We assumed that 20% of beds were occupied by patients who could be better cared for outside hospital (a conservative assumption); that actual acute bed numbers should be inflated by 10% to take account of the patients currently having to endure treatment in distant hospitals because no bed was available, and we also assumed that a safe level for bed occupancy is 85%. With these new assumptions, we ran the model again, using census data to predict desirable levels of provision.

Our next step was to apply unit costs to both the predicted levels of each service required, and the actual costs of the existing levels of provision, enabling comparisons to be drawn.

Actual costs

It emerges that actual costs, expressed per 100,000 population at risk, are much greater for hospital services in inner London (£3.6M/100K than for outer London (£1.9M/100K); while residential costs were more closely comparable (£2.8M/100K inner, £2.1M/100K outer). We found wide variation between boroughs in the costs associated with provision, especially marked in outer London (Johnson et al., 1997, p. 317).

Actual versus predicted costs

When actual costs are compared with the costs predicted by the MINI, an interesting finding emerges: only in less deprived areas such as Brent, Richmond, Barnet and Bexley are the costs of actual provision fairly close to costs predicted by the MINI, whereas in deprived areas such as Camden, Lambeth, East London and Ealing actual costs are well below the levels predicted by the MINI.

The comparison of estimated need and actual provision shows that acute beds are one of the categories where variation appears greatest between areas, but overall, both inner and outer London emerge as having substantially fewer acute beds than the model predicts. For medium and for local secure provision, both inner and outer London emerge as having overall more provision than predicted—this is the case for most inner city areas, whilst the picture in outer London is mixed. The excess is greater for medium secure beds, again raising a question about whether the current balance between these two types of provision is the correct one.

The shortage of acute beds might conceivably contribute to this apparent excess provision. However, a more likely explanation may be that this is one of the categories for which assuming a linear relationship between deprivation and need for services is most flawed. In most of the deprived inner city areas, use of secure provision is at a high level regardless of local level of acute bed use, whereas some of the more affluent areas are using no or minimal quantities of this provision.

For 24-hour staffed and day-staffed and lower supported provision, the almost uniform picture across inner and outer London is of an apparent excess of the former and deficit of the latter. In outer London the apparent surplus of 24-hour staffed places is close in extent to the apparent deficit at lower levels of support, whilst in inner London the apparent shortfall of lower support places is about 1.5 times the apparent excess of 24-hour staffed accommodation. In summary, our results show that there are considerable shortfalls of all types of in-patient and residential care throughout the capital, and Table 2.2 shows the extent of these deficits for each local borough.

TABLE 2.2
Estimates of Shortfall of In-Patient Beds and Residential Accommodation in Inner London Boroughs

Borough	*Acute Beds*	*24-hour staffed*	*Low Support*
Camden	5	nk	52
Greenwich	17	33	−167
Hackney	16	148	16
Hammersmith	16	88	68
Islington	55	2	58
Kensington	3	72	0
Lambeth	63	16	−47
Lewisham	50	100	48
Southwark	40	54	4
Tower Hamlets	3	70	36
Wandsworth	70	26	76
Westminster	53	14	20
TOTAL	438	623	155

THE FUNCTIONING OF COMMUNITY MENTAL HEALTH SERVICES IN LONDON

In addition to the survey of residential and in-patient care, the King's Fund Report on London's Mental Health also gathered data on the functioning of community mental health services. While full details are published in the Johnson et al. (1997) report, we summarise the main findings here.

1. London's mental health services appear to be in transition towards a community-based model. Elements in establishing community services which require no major initial expenditure, such as sectorisation and organising staff into multidisciplinary teams, have largely taken place. However, in many areas, community premises for service delivery are not as yet available.

2. The general hospital A & E department still has a central place in emergency service delivery, particularly out of hours, despite some service delivery at community sites during office hours.

3. In some parts of the city, but most community service provision is still limited to office hours.

4. In most London catchment areas, acute home-based treatment services are not yet sufficiently highly developed for it to seem realistic to expect them to constitute an adequate substitute for admission. In some less deprived areas, acute day hospital response is sufficiently swift and available for it to appear likely that some patients can be diverted from admission from this facility—this is not generally the case in more deprived areas. Particularly in more deprived areas, CPN and social worker allocation appear too slow for the community service to be readily capable of a response which diverts admission. Thus overall our data suggest that in most parts of London community care has not yet developed to a point where it is likely often to be an adequate alternative to the acute ward.

5. For most major aspects of care, there are very significant shortages and delays in many parts of London, so that few areas are likely to be available to deliver reliably the comprehensive 'spectrum of care' recommended in policy documents.

6. For most service types, there is great variation between trusts in availability. Londoners in different parts of the metropolis are likely to be experiencing very different supplies of major services. A small minority of London's trusts do appear to be succeeding in delivering most major elements in care without serious delays and shortages arising.

7. There are also large variations in service availability within trusts. This draws attention to a need for researchers and planners to assess services in a detailed sector-by-sector way, as the view at the level of whole trusts will miss many such variations. It also raises the question of whether an unforeseen consequence of sectorisation may be an increase in inequity—prior to sectorisation, most services within a district or trust catchment area would presumably have been available to most residents, whereas now some small areas seem to experience great shortages of important services, despite their availability elsewhere in the catchment area.

IMPLICATIONS FOR LONDON'S MENTAL HEALTH

Is London different from other British cities?

London is found to share problems with other large cities in England, but to possess these problems in somewhat greater degree: the problems are especially marked in deprived inner city areas, where rates for psychotic illness—especially in younger males—are rising, rates are higher than those in the suburbs, there are high rates of mentally disordered offenders, and high rates of drug dependency and alcohol abuse. London has 22% more admissions to psychiatric beds per thousand population at risk than other cities; more single, divorced and widowed patients than elsewhere; more admissions from ethnic minorities; 4.2% more patients with a diagnosis of schizophrenia; more admissions with drug dependency; and more discharges to residential facilities in the community.

Are the problems due to the health purchasing authorities?

We found that London's purchasing authorities were spending more of their total health budgets on mental health: 18.6% in London, *vs* 12.8% in other deprived cities. Yet London seems to be at a disadvantage for four reasons: it has to deal with more admissions/1000; it has to pay for more mentally disordered offenders (and these are very expensive); it has more patients with a dual diagnosis of drug problems and psychosis (and these are twice as expensive as either condition on its own); and the shortage of acute beds means that patients are paid for in expensive private hospitals. Thus although the total allocations of money to purchasers take account of census indicators of social deprivation, they probably do not take sufficient account of them, and London purchasers have to manage on relatively

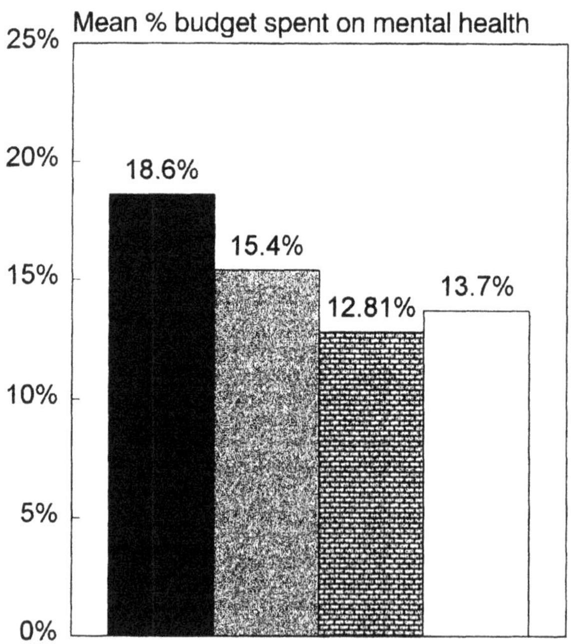

FIG. 2.5. Proportion of total health budget spent on mental health. ■, inner deprived London; ▩, mixed status London; ▤, high status London; □, inner deprived—not London.

worse budgets than their opposite numbers elsewhere. Thus, there is a substantial shortfall in cash support which is especially marked in the most deprived areas. Figure 2.5 shows the average proportion of total health authority budget spent on mental health in each geographical group.

LONDON'S FUTURE MENTAL HEALTH

Faced with these major challenges (summarised in Fig. 2.6), London's mental health system is unlikely to change for the better unless the new government makes some dramatic changes to the assumptions that underlie resource allocations to deprived inner cities across the country, and allow capital building programmes to start to provide the structures in which mental health professionals can work and users of the services can receive help. There is also a need to recruit more staff to work in the mental health service, and to consider other solutions if this turns out to be impossible. These include a greater use of volunteers, and of less intensively trained paid staff to carry out mental health work.

The new government also needs to consider ways of eliminating the

The hospital system cannot cope with high levels of demand:

- Bed occupancy rates as high as 125%, getting worse.
- Delays and long journeys for admission.
- In-patient beds being used inefficiently.
- Many assaults, sexual harassment on wards.
- High threshold for admission.
- A&E departments used during the night.
- Shortages of staff of all kinds; low morale.

The community services are characterised by:

- Lack of 24-hour residential places.
- Long delays for all community services.
- Ten-fold variation in low support accommodation.
- 24-hour community services almost entirely absent.
- Home treatment rarely available.
- Little day care; employment schemes.
- Ethnic minority services scanty.
- London's primary care services significantly worse than other large cities.

FIG. 2.6. Major challenges facing London's mental health services.

divide between health and social services expenditures, so that each locality receives a single mental health budget, adjusted to take account of social deprivation, out of which it can provide the most cost-effective forms of treatment, and the recent Turnberg review of London's health services reinforces these points (Department of Health, 1997, 1998). At present, much money is wasted keeping patients in expensive hospital beds, and sending others to expensive beds at sometimes great distance from their homes. We need minimum acceptable standards for waiting times, for bed occupancy rates, and for waits for community placements. Desirable practices—like supported tenancies, and permanent tenancies with varying levels of support, need to be actively encouraged. We need further development of services supporting carers, and to provide training for carers of mentally ill elderly.

Finally, there remains a need for further research: how many admissions could be prevented if 24-hour nursing were available in the community? Why are rates for psychosis rising among young males? How can cultural sensitivity training best be given, to produce a service more capable of providing a satisfactory service to ethnic minorities? How can the service best recruit and train staff? The King's Fund hopes to encourage our new government to engage in a constructive dialogue about improving the health care received by Londoners.

REFERENCES

Davidge, M., Elias, S., Jayes, B., Wood, K., & Yates, J. (1993). *Survey of English mental illness hostels: Prepared for the Mental Health Task Force.* Health Services Management Centre, University of Birmingham.

Davies, S., Thornicroft, G., Leese, M., Higginbotham, A., & Phelan, M. (1996). Ethnic differences in risk of compulsory admission among representative cases of psychosis in London. *British Medical Journal, 312*, 533–537.

Department of Health (1997). *The Future of London's Health Services* (*The Turnberg Report*). London: HMSO.

Department of Health (1998). *Health services in London. A strategic review.* London: Department of Health.

Glover, G.R. (1996). The Mental Illness Needs Index (MINI). In G. Thornicroft, & G. Strathdee (Eds) *Commissioning Mental Health Services.* London: HMSO.

HMSO (1994). House of Commons Health Committee. *Memorandum from the Department of Health on Public Expenditure on Health and Personal Social Services.* London: HMSO.

Jarman, B., Hirsch, S., White, P., & Driscoll, R. (1992). Predicting psychiatric admission rates. *British Medical Journal, 304*, 1146–1151.

Johnson, S., & Lelliot, P. (1997). Mental health services in London: Evidence from research and routine data. In: S. Johnson et al. (op. cit). pp. 167–192.

Johnson, S., Ramsay, R., Thornicroft, G., Brooks, L., Lelliot, P., Peck, E., Smith, H., Chisholm, D., Audini, B., Knapp, M., & Goldberg, D. (1997). *London's Mental Health.* London: Kings Fund.

King, M., Coker, E., Leavey, G., Hoare, A., & Johnson-Sabine, E. (1994). Incidence of psychotic illness in London: Comparison of ethnic groups. *British Medical Journal, 304*, 1115–1119.

Meltzer, H., Gill, B., Petticrew, M., & Hinds, K. (1995). *The prevalence of psychiatric morbidity among adults living in private households. OPCS surveys of psychiatric morbidity in Great Britain*. London: HMSO.

Office of Population Censuses and Surveys. (1993). *Mid year population estimates 1993*. London: HMSO Government statistical service.

Thornicroft, G. (1991). Social deprivation and rates of treated mental disorder: developing statistical models to predict psychiatric service utilisation. *British Journal of Psychiatry, 158*, 475–484.

CHAPTER THREE

Mental health services in Amsterdam

Aart H. Schene
University of Amsterdam, The Netherlands
Eric Hoffmann and Ad L.J. Goethals
APCP, Amsterdam, The Netherlands

THE CITY OF AMSTERDAM

Introduction

In this chapter we first give general information about Amsterdam's history, the population and housing, economy, culture and administration. Secondly, we describe some of the major social and health problems. The third theme is the history, transformation and the characteristics of Amsterdam's mental health services. We finish with a discussion of current issues and conclusions.

Short history

Amsterdam has been the capital of the Netherlands since 1806. Although the Houses of Parliament are located in The Hague, Amsterdam has been the leading Dutch metropolis since the 16th century. After the French period the economic revival started around 1870 when investments in the colonies gave the city the opportunity to become a centre for colonial trade. At the end of that century the city quickly expanded into an important industrial centre with shipyards, machine factories, and garment and foodstuff plants. After the Second World War many of the industrial activities disappeared. Today the city is mainly a centre for business, financial services, computer and medical technology.

Until the 1930s Amsterdam expanded in circles around the inner city. In 1935 the city council formulated a new conception of city planning. Further expansion was to be in the shape of loops, a plan implemented after the Second World War. In the 1950s new suburbs were successively added to the outskirts. Despite these expansions the housing shortage remained. In the early 1970s Amsterdam added one more large area, the Bijlmermeer, on the south-east side of the city.

During the last few decades people, mostly families with children, moved out to new towns, most miles away from the capital. They were replaced by youngsters, coming to the city to find a job or to study. During the last 15 years a lot of the city's housing has been renovated with the aim of encouraging people to live in the city. Wherever land became available, residential premises were built, especially for single people and couples without children.

Population and housing

In 1996 Amsterdam had a population of 722,350, including a figure of 316,228 (43.7%) single people. Of all inhabitants 19.9% are younger than 20 years, 13% are older than 65 years, while 6.3% are older than 75 years.

Amsterdam has a multi-ethnic population. Of all inhabitants 57.6% are Dutch. Ethnic minority groups are mainly people from Surinam (9.7%), Morocco (6.7%), Turkey (4.3%), Southern Europe (2.3%) and Antilles/Aruba (1.5%). Of the remaining 17.8%, 8.3% are from non-industrialised countries and 9.7% from industrialised countries.

The size of the city is 21,242 hectares. The number of housing units is 357,641: 11.4% are privately owned units, 32.9% privately rented and 54.6% rent-controlled units. In 1950 there were 835,834 inhabitants. Around 1960 the highest number of inhabitants, 870,000, was reached. The number dropped to the 722,350 mentioned, while the number of apartments rose to 357,641. Thus the average number of tenants per apartment has fallen from 3.77 in 1950 to 2.04 in 1996. In 1997 about 47,500 people were registered as looking for a place to live, two-thirds looking for a two-room apartment.

Economy and culture

The total number of people employed is 330,964. The employment 'top-10' includes commercial services and computer technology (41,192 employees), public health care and welfare (41,065), banks and insurance companies (28,580), wholesale and distributive trade (26,350), retail trade (25,780), government (25,453), school system (21,697), transport and services (16,492), hotels, restaurants and cafes (14,892) and professional organisations, culture and sports (13,008).

In 1996 some 83,000 people (20% of the 'working' population) were registered as unemployed (67% unemployed more than one year, 37% more than three years). Unemployment rates are unevenly distributed; for Dutch natives this percentage is 17, for immigrants from Southern-Europe 20%, for people from Surinam, the Antilles and Morocco about 40%, while for people from Turkey it goes up to 50%. A major problem is the 30% of the city's youngsters who leave secondary school without a diploma.

Amsterdam has two universities (35,600 students) and some colleges (28,200 students). It is one of Europe's leading tourist magnets and it has assimilated large numbers of newcomers from other cultures. The national airport Schiphol is one of the leading European airports. There is a stock exchange and options exchange and most banks have their headquarters in this city. The harbour is the second Dutch port. The city is the most important cultural centre in the Netherlands.

Administration

The City Council is the highest authority in Amsterdam and has 45 members. In 1990 Amsterdam completed the reorganisation of its administration. In addition to the central administration, the city is now divided into 16 districts of around 45,000 inhabitants. They have their own tasks, budget, officials and elected authorities like a District Chairman and Aldermen. The Sub-City Councils are responsible for housing, roads, public parks, indoor and outdoor public premises, education, public health, and the social and cultural facilities in their district.

City problems

Unemployment rates are especially high among ethnic minorities and young people. A lot of these youngsters have a low level of education, and criminality among them is relatively high. Also the percentage of elderly people (65^+) is relatively high, which also holds for the percentage of those living alone, not born in the Netherlands and for people with low education. One-third of the population is on some form of benefit.

An epidemiological study (Reijneveld, 1994) on the health of the Amsterdam people showed that in comparison with the Netherlands the total mortality, the perinatal mortality, the number of infectious diseases, the percentage unable to work, the percentage with chronic disabilities, the number of suicide attempts, and the percentage of hard drug addicts are significantly higher. AIDS has received a lot of special attention during the past decade. By April 1995 a total of 3488 of the 15 million Dutch people were diagnosed as having this illness. About half of them were living in Amsterdam.

Mobility is high. Many people at the beginning of their professional career leave Amsterdam. Because of the high mobility, the high percentage of single people, the increasing individualisation and loss of social networks, the problem of isolation and loneliness has increased considerably.

Criminality and safety in public life are high on the political agenda. The police, in addition to their everyday work, mainly focus on combatting juvenile crime, punishable acts affecting public safety, burglaries in homes, organised crime, local trade in drugs (with priority for nuisance caused by drug-related forms of crime and international drug trade), offences against the environment, and traffic safety.

Ethnic minorities

A quarter of the population belongs to one of the five minority groups mentioned. This figure is expected to rise to one-third by the year 2000. Almost half the pupils at the city's primary schools are now of non-Dutch descent. In some districts this percentage is significantly higher. In five to ten years 50% of the youngsters leaving school will be of 'foreign' descent. In the early 1980s a policy to help immigrants to assimilate was developed. This policy strongly focuses on the youth of today. The school system is still inadequately equipped for the multicultural population. Special attention is now devoted to elevating the disadvantages certain groups are still facing. The main policy is to bring about a coherent policy to reduce the educational handicaps of certain pupils, due to social, economic, or cultural factors.

Drug problems

There are about 6000 people in Amsterdam who use heroin and/or cocaine, 1500 are of Dutch descent and 1500 from Surinam, the Antilles or Morocco. About 3000 are from other countries in Europe, mainly Germany, Italy and Great Britain. The average age of the addicts rose from 26.8 in 1981 to 36.2 in 1995. About 1000 users regularly disturb the peace in the city. Often they are homeless, have no legal source of income, are mainly living in the city centre, and resort to crime to get money for their daily dose of drugs. In the inner city the law and order forces are mainly focused on this group: with surveillance, observation, arrests and the discouragement of concentration of users (see the section on addiction aid programmes later in the chapter).

Small quantities of soft drugs are sold at 'coffee shops'. Amsterdam has approximately 350 of these coffee shops, of which some 100 are also bars. The policy is focused on freezing these numbers and limiting the shops to certain parts of the city. It is forbidden to sell hard drugs there, to cause nuisance, or to sell to anyone under the age of 18. Advertising and transactions above five grams are forbidden. A customer can only buy for his own use. Failure to adhere to these conditions, or having a selling stock of more than 500 grams of soft drugs, leads to official measures, the most severe of which is the withdrawal of the coffee shop licence. Studies have shown that very few users go from soft to hard drugs, and the number of users has remained virtually the same since 1976.

MENTAL HEALTH SERVICES

To understand the history of Amsterdam's mental health services we consider in-patient services and community mental health services separately, and then try to explain how these two have attempted to reach each other.

History of the service, 1562–1980

1562–1930. The first 'madhouse' for people with mental disorders in Amsterdam was opened in 1562 and closed in 1792 (Vijselaar, 1997). From then a part of the Buitengasthuis, a general hospital located just outside the inner city area, became the only institution for people with mental disorders in Amsterdam. In 1840, when Amsterdam had 211,000 inhabitants, it gave places to 150 psychiatric patients.

In 1842 the Inspector of Health described this hospital as the most terrible, dirty and inhumane of the country. One year after this visit a large piece of land was bought 25 kilometres to the west of Amsterdam at the border of the dunes. In 1849 some 162 patients travelled by coach to the new mental hospital built there, which was called *Meerenberg*. This hospital had the whole province of North-Holland, including Amsterdam, as its catchment area. Hospital facilities for the city were the responsibility of the Province of North-Holland until 1991.

The number of patients rose from 500 in 1857, to 775 in 1866, and around 900 in 1882. The director of the hospital concluded by 1874 that this 'medical institution' had become a 'nursing home'. In 1885 a new building was opened for 400 patients which was occupied in about another 3 years, mainly because many Amsterdam patients hospitalised all over the Netherlands now returned to their 'city' hospital.

Because of Meerenberg's capacity problems the Buitengasthuis continued to admit psychiatric patients illegally. In 1883 it was decided to build a new hospital on the same grounds, the Wilhelminagasthuis. It was finished in 1893 and one of its three pavilions, *Pavilion III*, was meant for patients with mental diseases. Around 1900 the situation was again problematic and a new psychiatric hospital *Duin en Bosch* was built for the area to the north of Amsterdam.

In 1910 another psychiatric hospital, the *Valerius clinic*, was opened in Amsterdam. Both Pavilion III and the Valerius clinic later became University Clinics selecting the 'better' patients. Meerenberg increasingly became the mental hospital for the chronic and difficult patients of Amsterdam. In 1918 the reputation of Meerenberg had declined to such a low point that it was decided to change its name into the Provincial Hospital near Santpoort or just *'Santpoort'*.

1930–1960. In 1931 around 3000 patients from Amsterdam were hospitalised in about 40 different psychiatric hospitals all over the country, many of them in Santpoort, which had 1500 beds at that time (Amsterdam having 700,000 inhabitants). In that year the later well known psychiatrist Querido was given the task of visiting these patients, and to propose methods that could reduce the number of admissions. Querido (1935, 1968) developed the very first example world-wide of admission prevention by outreaching home visits. This independent social psychiatric service was a section of the Department of Mental Hygiene of the Amsterdam Municipal Health Service. The aim of this *'psychiatrie d'urgence'* was to reduce the number of admissions by providing pre-care, outreaching psychiatric emergency services and aftercare. Through this service the rising number of admissions, around 100 per year in the period 1926–1930, came to a standstill.

Other community mental health services began to develop in Amsterdam as well. In 1928 the first Dutch Medical Education Bureau was opened, aimed at the prevention of psychiatric disorders by diagnosing and treating children with mental problems. At the beginning of the Second World War the first Institute for Multidisciplinary Psychotherapy started, and at the end of this war the first Bureau for Personal and Family Counselling.

In the 1950s, community mental health care became partly organised along religious lines. In Amsterdam, for instance, the Protestant (1948) and Catholic Foundation (1950) for Mental Health each organised under one roof the different ambulatory organisations; a Medical Education Bureau, a Bureau for Personal and Family Counselling and a Social Psychiatric Service.

1960–1980. In the 1960s, ambulatory mental health services included four regionalised Medical Education Bureaux, two independent Bureaux for Personal and Family Counselling, the two multifunctional foundations on religious bases, and in particular for psychotherapy, an Institute for Multidisciplinary Psychotherapy and a Psychoanalytic Institute. There was also the already mentioned Department of Mental Hygiene of the Amsterdam Municipal Health Service. So services were organised according to different principles; religion, type of therapy and type of institution.

The 1960s saw the first ideas concerning non-denominational segregated ambulatory mental health care and sectorisation. Finally in 1972 on the national level the Dutch Association of Ambulatory Mental Health Care (NVAGG) was founded, followed in 1975 by its Amsterdam counterpart (AVAGG). Using the American Community Mental Health Care Centres as an example, both associations aimed at organising integrated multidisciplinary ambulatory mental health care, including social psychiatry, in *Regional Institutes for Community Mental Health Care* (RIAGG) for all age groups. In contrast to the American example, these RIAGGs did not have beds nor day hospital facilities, nor any formal relation with psychiatric hospitals. In fact they were organised to be a strong counterforce against the mental hospitals, which in that decade were seen as powerful and conservative institutions.

Regarding these mental hospitals, opposition increased in the 1970s with the Amsterdam client movement as one of the leading powers, inspired by authors like Goffman, Laing, Szasz, Basaglia, Marcuse and Foucault. There was also the beginning of a critical atmosphere within the hospitals. Partly as a reaction to this opposition, mental hospitals began a process of expansion, modernisation, differentiation, and democratisation. Financial limitations were relatively scarce. For the psychiatric hospitals this not only meant adding new functions, but also a renewal of old facilities. After many protests regarding the very bad conditions in long-stay wards, the Dutch government in 1977 started the nationwide project 'Re-housing Psychiatry', aimed at the rebuilding of the old wards on the same grounds.

In 1974 Santpoort opened a special unit for acute admissions and a resocialisation unit for 360 patients. The years that followed made clear that the optimism about resocialisation, about reintegrating patients back from the dunes into Amsterdam, was in many cases too high. In 1979 the 360–bed resocialisation unit was divided into one unit for long-stay patients and a resocialisation unit. It was also realised that a substantial number of the patients would not leave the hospital; 70% were already older than 60, and 50% older than 70 years. In 1980 a new 340 bed unit was built for chronic and psychogeriatric patients.

Strong opposition: 1980–1985

Financial arguments entered the health care discussion in the early 1980s. The Province of North-Holland had too much hospital capacity, while the capital itself had a limited number of psychiatric beds—the two psychiatric university clinics with their selective admission policy. The idea of bringing Santpoort back to Amsterdam, born in the early '70s, was revitalised. In

1980 the government gave Santpoort permission to build a 350 bed psychiatric hospital in Amsterdam on the grounds of the Wilhelminagasthuis. As a prelude, Santpoort took over Amsterdam's crisis centre and the centre for day treatment in 1981. Plans for building new hospital facilities in the city were frozen in 1982 due to a nationwide discussion about a moratorium on new hospitals, very much influenced by new ideas about the organisation of mental health care in the capital.

Hospital and community care. The situation in Amsterdam in the early 1980s was complicated. The city's mental hospital Santpoort, still far away, was in a process of renewal. There were ideas and first initiatives about coming back to Amsterdam, but the building of new hospitals in the city was blocked. At the same time the number of admissions was growing, even more so for the percentage of involuntary admissions—the beginning of the 'revolving door' phenomenon.

On the other hand, the field of community mental health care was fragmented. These services were not enthusiastic about a formal relation with the hospitals due to their fear of stigmatisation of their own patient population, mostly people with less severe psychiatric problems. Besides there were powers in favour as well as against regionalisation. The Institute for Multidisciplinary Psychotherapy and the Psychoanalytic Institute, for instance, did not want to regionalise their services.

Following nationwide developments it was decided in 1978 that with regard to RIAGGs Amsterdam also should be sectorised. It took another three years before it was decided to start five RIAGGs. In a difficult process almost all the different ambulatory services were reorganised into five RIAGGs. These institutes brought together professionals from different theoretical and religious backgrounds, as well as professionals who used to work for patients of different age groups. This difficult integration process took many years. As a result community mental health care became available for every inhabitant of the capital.

The Department of Mental Hygiene was also opposed against regionalisation. This community service had frequent contacts with Santpoort and more or less served the same type of patients. Both services by the end of the 1960s planned to build a social psychiatric institution in Amsterdam. This 350-bed institution would have had the whole city as its catchment area and would have included acute admission wards until then located at the Santpoort hospital. These plans were never realised.

Of all the ambulatory services two continued to work on the city level; the Psychoanalytic Institute and a part of the Department of Mental Hygiene, which in the evening and night-time hours still organised the city-wide crisis intervention service. In 1994 this service was closed. From then acute psychiatric services were organised on a regional level.

City and province. In the years 1982 to 1984 relations were strained but the Client Movement was most successful in organising sufficient political support for its new ideas about service delivery. Inspired by countries such as Italy, progressive forces, young scientists, professionals and clients started to work together with one common target; to break down the restrictive, dehumanising and isolating aspects of psychiatry. This meant, among other things, isolation rooms, electroshock therapy, and stigmatising treatments, all represented by 'the mental hospital'.

In 1982 young scientists presented the document 'The Amsterdam way to a new style mental health care system' (van der Poel & van Haaster, 1982). Their ideas were translated into a 'Note considering integral management of mental health care in Amsterdam', which was passed by the City Council unanimously in 1984, a date that can formally be seen as the start of the Transformation Process. It was of great importance that this note was endorsed by the province, and that the Provincial Deputy for Health and the Amsterdam Alderwoman for Health could agree on a protocol describing the principles and structure of the mental health transformation process.

In 1983 the government decided that Santpoort should have full responsibility for the Amsterdam region. Psychiatric hospitals no longer had the opportunity to be renewed and rebuilt on their original locations. They now had to decentralise, bringing back services to the places where people were living.

Transformation: 'The Amsterdam Model'

To develop an integrated system of mental health care Amsterdam was divided into three—and not as for the RIAGGs five—regions. Three committees began their work in 1984 (Gersons, van de Graaf, Rijkschroeff, & Schrameyer, 1992); (1) a Steering Committee for the co-ordination of the whole process, (2) an Advisory Committee of independent specialists advising the Steering Committee on specific issues, and (3) a Project Committee for each of the three regions. Between 1984 and 1986 the Advisory Committee produced six recommendations, presented in 1987 as a concluding report entitled *The Amsterdam Model* (Advisory Committee Mental Health Care Amsterdam, 1987).

Also in 1984 the collaboration of progressive forces, including some clients, was transformed into the *Platform for Mental Health Care.* It received a subsidy from the municipal authorities which was spent on research. Between 1984 and 1989 reports were published regarding *The future of ambulatory mental health care in Amsterdam*, *Primary care*, *Partial hospitalisation, new style; a social psychiatric approach*, and *Supporting client participation in mental health care.*

Transformation. To summarise the principles, nowadays well known in community psychiatry, that have been critical for the Amsterdam transformation process we look at the client, service and service delivery levels (Gersons et al., 1982; Schene, Henderson, Knudsen, Rijkschroeff, & Thornicroft, 1992).

Considering clients:

1. Clients and client organisations will have influence on all the different levels.
2. Service delivery is individualised, needs-based and tailor made.
3. Clients stay as much as possible within their own living circumstances.
4. Stigmatisation and marginalisation are opposed.
5. The repressive function of psychiatry is opposed.
6. Chronic mentally ill, migrants and women are prioritised.

Considering services:

1. Services are small scale.
2. Services are regionalised and evenly distributed over the city.
3. Only a minimum of services are organised on city level.
4. Collaboration between primary care and mental health care.
5. Emphasis on out-patient and semimural services.
6. Integration of ambulatory, semimural and in-patient services.
7. Admissions to in-patient services are minimised by an outreach approach, partial hospitalisation and time-out facilities.
8. Segregation of living and treatment.
9. Differentiation in housing accommodation.
10. Emphasis on rehabilitation.
11. Continuity of care.
12. Development of community support systems.

Considering service delivery: the city will be divided into three regions, of around 200,000 inhabitants each. Each region offers comprehensive and integrated mental health care including:

1. Ambulatory district teams: outreaching and offering social psychiatric care regardless of where patients are staying.
2. Social Psychiatric Service Centres; clinical crisis interventions, short treatments, either using in-patient or preferably day treatment services, a maximum of 40 beds.
3. Hotel accommodation: for patients that normally live on their own but temporarily need more protection or safety.
4. A differentiated system of sheltered living accommodation.

5. Day care and rehabilitation services.

Mental health service evaluation

There has never been a thorough and well-designed evaluation of Amsterdam's transformation process. However, a lot of smaller projects have been conducted, which taken together offer information about different aspects of this process.

In 1993 a report was published called *The Amsterdam Model halfway* (Janssen, 1993). It is an evaluation of the implementation of ideas underlying the transformation process, based on about 250 documents considering mental health services (mostly research reports) and on 52 interviews with key figures. In 1992 a Visiongroup started to evaluate the transformation of Amsterdam's mental health care on the actual provision of services. It had to formulate new principles according to which further developments could be checked. In 1993 they published *Starting points for mental health care in Amsterdam in the Nineties.* Both reports were translated into the Regional Vision on Amsterdam Mental Health Care in the Nineties.

Santpoort's return to Amsterdam: 1986–1996

Decentralisation was necessary, but breaking Santpoort hospital up into small units, or even ideas about integration and fusion with other mental health care services in Amsterdam, was at that time not acceptable. In 1986 the Board of Directors stated that Santpoort could only contribute by a transfer to Amsterdam of some of the hospital's services. The hospital continued to vacillate between moving to Amsterdam and staying in the dunes. In 1986 a unit for psychomotor therapy was built on the hospital grounds, and as late as 1990 a new kitchen was opened, both for a population of 1200 patients. In 1989 the Province decided to privatise the hospital. In 1991 the hospital was officially taken over by two new organisations; Frederik van Eeden Foundation and the Psychiatric Hospital Amsterdam. In 1992 these finally decided to return all—not only acute—Santpoort services to Amsterdam within a ten year period. With this decision the three regions got their own 'mental hospital'; *Frederik van Eeden Foundation* (East/South-East), *Psychiatric Hospital Amsterdam* (Centre/Old-West/North), and the *Amsterdam Psychiatric Centre* (South/New-West), a fusion of the Valerius clinic and a residential service (J.C. de Keijzer), both already located in Amsterdam.

To understand Santpoort's return we consider services for long-term patients and the services for acute admissions separately.

Residential services. The Advisory Committee stated that living accommodation for long-term patients should be small scale, in the neighbourhood where patients (used to) live and situated as much as possible in normal houses. In 1986 Santpoort made plans for the return to Amsterdam of the first groups of long-term patients. Half a year earlier than expected, forced by heating facilities that broke down in the old wards during wintertime, 36 long-term patients moved to flats in the Bijlmermeer. In this sheltered living project ('*Kempering*'), patients lived in 1–4-person apartments on the lowest layer of big flats. There was a nursing office, an apartment for other staff members, a day care centre and a kitchen. Within half a year 12 patients returned to Santpoort. However the project demonstrated that some patients were able to live more independent lives than was expected when they were hospitalised. In 1987 a second group of 74 chronic patients moved to a building in Amsterdam (*Surinameplein*) close to the centre. These patients started to live in groups of 15, with a sitting room, washing and toilet facilities for their own use.

Both projects, *Kempering* and *Surinameplein,* were evaluated (Duurkoop, 1995). In comparison to their 'old' lives patients showed less symptomatology, better functioning, more social contacts, less use of seclusion, less beds on closed units and the same amount of medication. They were more satisfied, although integration within the neighbourhood was not successful. Rehabilitation should get far more attention, it was concluded.

In 1984 Amsterdam had 365 sheltered living homes, mostly psychiatric nursing homes with 24–hour nursing, owned by Regional Institutes of Sheltered Living, organisations independent of mental hospitals. Between 1984–1993 the number of sheltered living homes rose by 390 to 755; 268 places created by substitution of Santpoort long-stay beds and 122 places created by Regional Institute of Sheltered Living. The 268 were 200 below the 480–target for a 5–year period. Another target not realised was the percentage of places situated in normal houses, 38 in 1993 instead of 70. Presently the former Santpoort still houses 300 older and more difficult long-term patients. The hospital will finally close in 2001.

Acute services: social psychiatric service centres. For the acute admissions a Social Psychiatric Service Centre (offering crisis interventions, short treatments, either using in-patient or preferably day treatment services) should be organised for a population of about 120,000. The first one (Centre/Old-West; 76 in-patient/day-patient places) opened in 1988. The 'return to Amsterdam' was not well prepared. The starting period was a difficult one, with suicides of patients and a lot of sick-leave amongst the personnel (Cohen & Sanders, 1995). Dekker (1996) evaluated this first centre. In comparison with Santpoort, patients were referred at an earlier stage of decompensation, admissions were less urgent and more during day time hours. Patients were less secluded, there was less violence, patients were more satisfied and the percentage of day-hospital treatment was significantly higher than in Santpoort. In terms of length of stay, symptom reduction or functioning there were no differences.

In 1994 Santpoort's admission ward closed and the second and third centre were opened in Amsterdam-North (82 in-patient/day-patient places) and Amsterdam-East (69 places). Other centres are in preparation in the regions South-East (64 places) and South/New-West (60 places). The one planned for the city centre has been cancelled.

In conclusion acute services will be organised in five Social Psychiatric Service Centres, each for a region of 100–120,000 inhabitants. Their capacity is 60–70 beds each, including about 20–30% day hospital places. They are successful in substituting in-patient for day-patient care. The original target to limit length of stay to a maximum of three months was not reached, partly because the continuity of care into residential services stagnates. The centres certainly changed the geographical distance between house and hospital. In 1995 74% of all admissions were within the region where the patient was living. The centres are criticised because they still function too much as small hospitals, with not enough attention paid to ambulatory mental health care, being a form of trans-institutionalisation instead of de-institutionalisation. The transformation process has been successful in implementing these centres, but they have become too dominant. Social psychiatric approaches still have to be developed in a more stringent way. Continuity of care and outreach require far more attention, especially in relation to RIAGGs.

Day care centres

Before 1985 only three day care centres were available, all controlled by independent foundations. Between 1985 and 1993 nine new centres were opened (including a Fountain House clubhouse), most of them in organisational terms connected to a psychiatric hospital, RIAGG or sheltered living service. Together they offer about 3500 half-day units (morning/afternoon) of day care per week. However, for a total of about 8500 estimated long-term psychiatric patients living in Amsterdam this seems insufficient.

Client participation

In the early 1990s the organisation of client influence and participation changed. The Platform for Mental Health Care (see 'Transformation: 'The Amsterdam Model'', above) slowly lost its political power. The Dutch health care system and the Department of Health discovered 'the client' as a new party. Competition entered the health care system. Clients now became health care consumers whose demands had to be clarified and whose satisfaction had to be measured. For the government a reduction in costs became increasingly important, and critical client organisations were seen as being of great potential help in this process. The LPCP (National Patient Consumers Platform) started in 1989, and the APCP (Amsterdam Patient Consumers Platform) in 1990. This organisation is a collaboration of all health care consumer organisations, each with a particular section, in our case mental health care.

HEALTH CARE IN AMSTERDAM: FACTS

All mental health care (except psychiatric departments of general hospitals) is under one type of insurance, which for budgetary reasons, makes a distinction between intra-, semi- and extramural care. The intramural compartment includes organisations or institutions by law defined as general psychiatric hospitals or addiction clinics. The semimural compartment includes Regional Institutes for Sheltered Living, organising a variety of living accommodation. The extramural compartment includes the Regional Institutes for Ambulatory Mental Health Care (RIAGG), psychiatrists and ambulatory addiction services. Of the total annual budget intra-, semi- and extramural respectively get 71.2%, 5.7% and 23.1%.

Ambulatory (RIAGGs) and out-patient

Most RIAGGs have three sections; children/adolescents, adults and 60^+. Their target population overlaps with that of the out-patient departments of psychiatry connected to psychiatric hospitals or departments of psychiatry of general or academic hospitals. Amsterdam has five RIAGGs (North, East, South-East, South/New-West and Centre/Old-West). They have a total of about 45,000 new clients a year. The 7-day, 24–hour crisis intervention services are part of the RIAGG remit.

There are four out-patient departments of psychiatry for adults, each connected to a Social Psychiatric Service Centre, and three connected to psychiatric departments of general/academic hospitals. The exact number of new patients here is not known (estimated: 9000). Psychiatrists working independently from services have about 3000 new patients a year.

Specialists and hospitals

Amsterdam has two academic hospitals (1833 beds) and five general hospitals (2245 beds; 311 per 100,000 inhabitants). Academic hospitals have a catchment area much larger than Amsterdam. The total number of medical specialists *living* in Amsterdam is 1409, the number of residents is 719. Of these 2128 some 322 are psychiatrists or psychiatric residents (15.1%). The number of psychiatrists as well as other disciplines working just for the Amsterdam population is not known.

For each region a psychiatric hospital offers differentiated services; in-patient, day-patient, out-patient, residential and home care or other care innovations:

1. East/South-East (200,000 inhabitants, Frederik van Eeden Foundation):
   133 in-patient/day-patient places
   154 living accommodation/care at home
   73 psychogeriatric clinics
   89 in-patient (still in Santpoort).
2. Centre/Old-West/North (260,000 inhabitants, Psychiatric Hospital Amsterdam):
   158 in-patient/day-patient places
   64 living accommodation
   98 day treatment places
   194 in-patient (still in Santpoort).
3. South/New-West (240,000 inhabitants, Psychiatric Centre Amsterdam):
   141 in-patient/day-patient places
   166 long-term/living accommodation
   90 day treatment places.

Not regionalized and with a bigger catchment area:

1. Psychiatric Department Academic Medical Centre:
   60 in-patient and 34 day-patient places.
2. Psychiatric Department General Hospital St Lucas:
   30 in-patient and 16 day-patient places.
3. Jellinek centre (Addiction):
   211 in-patient places.
4. Nursing home for psychogeriatric patients:
   360 beds.

Amsterdam in 1995 had 1502 in-patient units counted as beds. Of these 432 were for acute services (in-patient/day-patient in Social Psychiatric Service Centres), 188 for day treatment, 73 for psychogeriatrics, 384 for living accommodation and 283 were long-term beds still in Santpoort.

For the year 2000 the following number of in-patient places per 1000 are allowed by law:

1. Psychiatric hospital and psychiatric department of general or academic hospital: 1.4 (1152 in-patient places).
2. Categorical psychiatric hospital: 0.17 (130 in-patient places).
3. Free margin: 0.20 (165 in-patient places).
4. Big city raise: 0.13 (107 in-patient places).

The number of 1502 has to be decreased to 1259 (1107+107) in the year 2000. This means a reduction of 243 in-patient places. The free margin will be used for child and adolescent psychiatry, addiction services and care innovation projects.

Residential services

Three types are distinguished:

1. Those for patients whose selfcare is moderate or sufficient. These are administered by the Regional Institutes for Sheltered Living (487 places).
2. Psychiatric living accommodation (384 places), for patients in need of some form of nursing. These are substituted psychiatric hospital beds, still budgeted and calculated as in-patient places.
3. Three social boarding houses (170 beds); set up in the last few years for homeless people with psychiatric disorders.

General practitioners

The total number of general practitioners is 479 (1507 inhabitants per general practitioner; 67.3 general practitioners per 100,000 inhabitants). The density of general practitioners in the different districts varies greatly. It is increasingly difficult to get general practitioners for the old, low income districts.

Municipal health service

The core of the city's public health care is the Municipal health service (GG&GD) founded in 1901 to replace the obsolete system of doctors for the poor. After the Second World War the service expanded into a modern department for collective/preventive health care. It combats infectious diseases, has ambulant services, provides health care for Amsterdam youngsters from 0 to 19 years, and is responsible among others for the police physicians, Aids-research, care for the homeless, drug addiction facilities, tuberculosis testing and care of the medical environment. The service advises city authorities on the health aspect of municipal policies.

Addiction aid programmes

A number of addiction aid programmes have been developed. The methadone programme of the municipal health service provides addicts with a daily dose of methadone. Through a mobile dispensary, a number of stationary ones, and from some general practitioners, half of the approximately 6000 hard drug addicts receive their methadone. The programme enables drug addicts to continue to function within society in a more or less normal fashion. To reduce the spread of AIDS and hepatitis B there are ten sites where addicts can exchange used needles for new ones free of charge. Only 40% of the addicts inject drugs. Most of them inhale.

In 1989 the 'street junkie project' was launched for the 1000 users who regularly disturb city-life. If criminal drug-users have four run-ins with the police within a 12–month period, they get a choice; either serve the entire sentence for their crimes without probation, or submit to treatment to help them stop using drugs. If they do not complete the entire treatment, they have to serve their entire prison sentence.

Miscellaneous

The number of dentists is 480 (1504 inhabitants/dentist), the number of pharmacies is 86, the number of social nurses is 187 and the number of beds for the mentally handicapped is 418.

MENTAL HEALTH SERVICE UTILISATION

Adding all admissions to in-patient, day-patient and sheltered living accommodation, the admission rate/1000 inhabitants is 6.04/year for Amsterdam and 4.68 for the Netherlands: 29% higher for Amsterdam. When the number of new clients per year in the RIAGGs are added this percentage rises to 43%. For the RIAGGs the percentage of new clients per 1000 in 1989 was 15.4 for men and 20.5 for women. For the Netherlands these figures were 12.0 and 14.7. More interesting is the total number of contacts/client; 8.2 for the Netherlands and 16.8 for Amsterdam.

The number of admissions for schizophrenia per 1000 inhabitants in the age group 20–34 years is 0.6 for the Netherlands and 2.4 for Amsterdam. For the category Other Psychoses the number is also significantly higher (0.45 *vs* 0.90). Ethnic groups differ significantly, as shown in Table 3.1.

Ethnic minority groups are hospitalised less often, if admitted more often as involuntary, more often with a diagnosis of schizophrenia, and the length of stay is shorter in comparison with Dutch people.

TABLE 3.1
Percentage of the Total Population, the Percentage of all Admissions (2.883) and the Total Number of Admissions per 1000 Inhabitants

Ethnic Group	*% of Population*	*% of Admissions*	*Admissions/1000*
Dutch	58.1	76.3	5.24
Surinam	9.6	7.5	3.13
Antilles	1.5	1.2	3.43
Turkey	4.3	1.5	1.39
Morocco	6.5	3.7	2.29
South-Europe	2.2	0.9	1.61
Other industrialised	8.1	3.7	1.85
Other non-industrialised	9.7	5.0	2.06

Involuntary admissions. The first years of the transformation process (1985–1991) showed a 44% decline in the number of involuntary admissions. This trend has changed over the past years; the percentage of patients involuntarily admitted rose over the years 1992 to 1995 from 6.1% to 15.9. Considering only admissions shorter than 6 months, percentages of involuntary admissions were 1993: 12%, 1994: 18%, and 1995: 21%. The number of involuntary admissions per 1000 inhabitants is 0.60 in Amsterdam and 0.31 in the Netherlands.

Regionalisation. The percentage of people using mental health care in their own region rose from 61% in 1992, to 64% in 1993, to 67% in 1994. Of all Amsterdam people that had to be admitted 10.1% were admitted outside the city, mostly people in the age group 20 to 34 years.

Costs. The Insurance Company has conducted a study on the development of costs for mental health care after the introduction of the Amsterdam Model. Between 1984 and 1989 they calculated a reduction of 4.5%, and they expected this reduction to increase to 7% in 1993. However, when mental health care costs per insured person are compared, the price for Amsterdam is 150% of the price in the Netherlands.

DISCUSSION AND FUTURE CHALLENGES

Ten years of care innovation in Amsterdam has changed much in the delivery of mental health services. Of course we should realise that during the last decades there have been among others major sociological, political, financial and technological changes. These have altered individual demands, needs and lifestyles, as well as interpersonal ways of behaviour, acceptance and support. Society has become more individualistic and less tolerant towards deviant behaviour. At the same time the percentage of people using ambulatory mental health care has increased tremendously during the last 15 years.

Since the start of the transformation process differentiation and decentralisation have been implemented. More individualised tailor-made care is possible now. However, although regionalisation has been successful, continuity of care has to be developed more rigorously. A major reason for stagnation on this point is that collaboration between services (RIAGG, out-patient departments, sheltered living, day care) is still low, let alone managerial and administrative integration or fusion between different services. For the near future this collaboration needs a strong emphasis otherwise principles of community psychiatry can not be implemented according to current standards.

One of the aims was to decrease the pushing-out or expulsion of psychiatric patients from the community. The transformation certainly has done a good job in counteracting these processes. There nevertheless is a growing group of people with psychiatric disorders who are not reached by mental health services. An important event took place in 1993 when a psychiatric patient living in a working-class quarter killed a child. This 'Vrolikstraat murder' initiated much discussion in the media about a failing mental health care system.

Santpoort's in-patient capacity has been relocated to Amsterdam as Social Psychiatric Service Centres, residential services, home care and nursing homes. To finance the return of those services still located in Santpoort to Amsterdam a further reduction of the total number of beds was necessary; 117 will be closed. Financial reserves are now available to start the building of new facilities in Amsterdam. Especially important is a further increase in the amount of living accommodation. Housing with flexible amounts of support, small scale in normal houses, are needed and very much preferred by clients.

Two types of services of the Amsterdam Model so far have not been realised; the social psychiatric district teams and the hotel accommodation. In theory the district teams were the core of the Amsterdam Model, outreaching, flexible and supportive. They should have offered a variety of treatment methods for a target population of about 50–70,000 people. The teams had to be composed of professionals from RIAGGs and Social Psychiatric Service Centres. Why did they fail? First it is not surprising that professionals connected to different types of services do not work together without coordination, and this is what has been lacking. Second, in the mid-1980s the RIAGGs were still in their infancy, trying to bridge the many differences between heterogeneous groups of professionals. They were not in need of another reorganisation. By law the RIAGGs got the task to offer outreaching acute and social psychiatric care, but they were not yet equipped for that task and their budgets were too low to offer it in such an intense way as intended for the district teams. The long history of opposition between psychiatric hospital, ambulatory services and Department of Mental Hygiene was not a good basis for a new joint task as the district teams. Last but not least these teams were also criticised by the clients which considered the teams as a further 'psychiatrising of society'.

The hotel accommodation was meant for those patients in need of some rest and support, temporarily not able to sleep in their own house or not having a house at all. Instead of this facility, partial hospitalisation has become very popular during the 1980s (Schene, van Lieshout, & Mastboom, 1986; Schene, van Lieshout, & Mastboom, 1988), in particular as an alternative for full time hospitalisation. If patients are admitted to a Social Psychiatric Service Centre they occupy a bed, but this does not necessarily mean they use it. If they want to sleep in the clinic, they can. If they are able to sleep at home, they do. They can always return to the clinic because their bed is vacant. Insurance companies pay for these 'beds' (some call them inflatable beds) although they know that they are occupied at night-time only for a certain percentage of nights. However, these services still very much have a psychiatric label. During the coming years experiments with time-out facilities for crisis situations are needed.

The Model has been criticised for its selectivity. It has been labelled a social psychiatric model which paid too little attention to youth (in particular adolescent psychiatry) as well as to psychotherapy, psychosocial problems, addiction services, severely handicapped patients, patients with double handicaps (somatic/psychiatric) and patients with severe behavioural disorders (aggressive/ forensic). The return of Santpoort to the capital was the great topic. Little attention has been paid to the several hundreds of long-term patients from Amsterdam hospitalised in psychiatric hospitals in other provinces than North-Holland. So far they are not incorporated in the calculations.

The process has also been criticised for being too much oriented on the organisation of (hospital) services, without realising that behind all these organisations professionals had to do the job. In particular the formation of the RIAGGs received far too little attention in the original ideas. The different types of services RIAGGs offer (e.g. 7-day, 24–hour crisis intervention, prevention, public mental health, consultations to public services) were not worked out in the Amsterdam Model. At the time the Model was designed, RIAGGs were in their infancy. Criticism of the psychiatric hospital structure of the 1970s was the driving force behind the Amsterdam Model, not a more modern one in which new developments were integrated. The dominance of organisational solutions also did not take into consideration the very difficult, conservative and limiting laws and regulations. New corporate bodies were mentioned as a solution to long-standing diverse interests. Only recently has such a body been created in one of the three regions (East/South-East).

One cannot blame the designers of the Model for having only limited knowledge about rehabilitation, which was also in its infancy at that time. However, further developments have shown the great importance and need for that type of service. Like elsewhere Social Psychiatric Service Centres, residential services and day care centres silt up with long-term users. What is needed is a very strong impulse towards the further development of rehabilitation techniques and practices in which consumer-run projects have to be emphasised.

Evaluations of the Model have recently enumerated groups of vulnerable people which need more attention: patients for a long period of their lives in need of psychiatric care and formerly hospitalised for many years, homeless people with severe psychiatric disorders, patients with a psychiatric and addiction disorder, patients from ethnic minorities, victims of sexual abuse or aggression, and young people with psychiatric problems. Most of these groups have become more pronounced during the last ten years. Special programmes have been developed but a lot more has to be done.

Much attention is given now to initiatives to reach those long-term patients who have great difficulty in matching the type of mental health care regularly offered. Care providers call them 'care avoiders'. In each region projects have been organised since 1993–94 to reach this group by active outreach strategies. They try to contact patients, help them with everyday problems, start rehabilitation and refer them to volunteers who help to build up a network. Some projects also are active in trying to work with the homeless mentally ill, in the (social) guest houses they stay in and on the streets; psychiatry takes to the streets, also in Amsterdam (Cohen, 1990). These initiatives are taken by the RIAGGs, sometimes by the decentralised psychiatric hospitals, and also by the former Department of Mental Hygiene, still responsible for public mental health.

In a dehospitalised system, mental health care can only be successful if it works together with other authorities, like housing associations, care for the homeless, (voluntary) work associations, community centres, legal advice centres and education. The main purpose of this 'flanking policy' is to organise a much larger safety net and more support for those vulnerable people constantly balancing on the border of society, sometimes causing nuisance and inconvenience for other people living in the neighbourhood. Safety Net & Advise, for instance, supports different district projects which have been called 'Extreme Nuisance'. Here a social psychiatric nurse, if necessary with a police officer, visits people who cause a lot of annoyance to their neighbours, and tries to find solutions.

Consumer participation needs more attention. Consumers have played an important role in the development of the Amsterdam Model, but their power and influence on the present services are far less pronounced. On the regional level, on health care policy, as well as in individual cases this influence should increase. Since 1996 the City of Amsterdam and the Insurance Company together finance a new way of client research, the Client Panel. By this method users of mental health services are interviewed by users, or they fill in questionnaires around a specific topic. Two reports have been published, one on Acute psychiatric care and one on Living Accommodation. The first one showed some major problems. Crisis intervention services have thresholds too high for many users. Each region needs a crisis intervention centre organised separately from psychiatric services. Although in organisational terms regionalisation is acceptable, users from all over the city must have the opportunity to use these centres.

CONCLUSION

We have described the development, transformation and current status of Amsterdam's mental health care services. It may be concluded that in the past ten years a lot of changes have been realised. The former psychiatric hospital Santpoort will finally be closed in 2001. All its services will have returned to Amsterdam, most of those in a decentralised and innovative way with a separation of acute and residential services.

However, currently there are some major concerns. First, although regionalisation has been implemented, the different mental health care services operating in a particular region are still not integrated into new corporate bodies. Here the great differences in historical backgrounds as well as budgets available for intra-, semi- and extramural services of course are a major obstacle. However a central coordinating and powerful body for the city as a whole has also been missing.

Second, it is evident that although Amsterdam has a lot of services there is nevertheless an increasing group of people with unmet needs. Most of them have a combination of severe psychosocial and psychological problems which do not match with existing health care and social services. Either these people, for whatever reason, do not want to be in contact with services, or the services are organised in such a rigid way that they do not meet the needs of these specific groups. Many of them are marginalised and excluded people who seem to be the victim of a society that is over-regulated and over-organised, and does not leave space for those who do not, or do not want to fit into these systems.

The challenges for the near future is to find a good balance between an increase of the overall quality of our society, in particular our cities, and an increase of the quality of life of those people who have disabilities or handicaps that make adaptation to the high demands and strict rules and regulations of such a society a hard job for them. They ask for deregulation, flexibility, solidarity, support, and special attention.

REFERENCES

Advisory Committee Mental Health Care Amsterdam. (1987). *Het Amsterdamse model (The Amsterdam Model): eindverslag van de adviesgroep Geestelijke Gezondheidszorg Amsterdam.* Amsterdam.

Cohen, D., & Sanders, H.E. (1995). Day-program-based treatment in the Amsterdam city centre. *International Journal of Social Psychiatry, 41*, 120–131.

Cohen, N.L. (1990). *Psychiatry takes to the streets. Outreach and crisis intervention for the mentally ill.* New York: Guilford Press.

Dekker, J. (1996). *Het Amsterdamse Sociaal Psychiatrisch Diensten Centrum (the Amsterdam Social Psychiatric Service Centre): een vergelijkend onderzoek naar een multi-functionele eenheid en de regulier 24-uurs zorg* [dissertation]. Amsterdam: Universiteit van Amsterdam.

Duurkoop, P. (1995). *Terug naar Amsterdam (Back to Amsterdam): longitudinaal onderzoek naar het functioneren van chronische patiënten in nieuwe woonsituaties.* Amsterdam: Frederik van Eeden Stichting.

Gersons, B.P.R., van de Graaf, W., Rijkschroeff, R., & Schrameyer, F. (1992). The mental health care transformation process: the Amsterdam experience. *International Journal of Social Psychiatry, 38*, 50–58.

Janssen, M. (1993). *Het Amsterdamse model halfweg (The Amsterdam Model Halfway): een tussenstand van de GGZ-hervormingen in de hoofdstad.* Utrecht: Nederlands centrum Geestelijke volksgezondheid.

Querido, A. (1935). Community mental hygiene in the city of Amsterdam. *Mental Hygiene, 19*, 177.

Querido, A. (1968). The shaping of community mental health care. *British Journal of Psychiatry*, 114, 293–302.

Reijneveld, S.A. (1994). *De gezondheid van de Amsterdammers (Health of the Amsterdam people): eindrapport van het project Gezondheidsprofiel Amsterdam.* Amsterdam: Gemeentelijke Geneeskundige en Gezondheidsdienst Amsterdam.

Schene, A.H., Henderson, J.H., Knudsen, H.C., Rijkschroeff, R., & Thornicroft, G. (1992). The evaluation of mental health care transformation in the cities of Europe. *International Journal of Social Psychiatry, 38*, 40–49.

Schene, A.H., van Lieshout, P., & Mastboom, J. (1986). Development and current status of partial hospitalization in the Netherlands. *International Journal of Partial Hospitalization, 3*, 237–246.

Schene, A.H., van Lieshout, P., & Mastboom, J. (1988). Different types of partial hospitalization programs: results from a nationwide study. *Acta Psychiatrica Scandinavica, 75*, 515–520.

van der Poel, E., & van Haaster, H. (1982). *Een Amsterdamse weg naar een GGZ nieuwe Stijl (The Amsterdam way to a new style mental health care system).* Amsterdam: SISWO.

Vijselaar, J. (Ed.) (1997). *Gesticht in de duinen (Asylum in the dunes): de geschiedenis van de provinciale psychiatrische ziekenhuizen van Noord-Holland van 1849 tot 1994.* Hilversum: Verloren.

CHAPTER FOUR

The city of Baltimore, USA: The Baltimore experience

Stephen T. Baron
Baltimore Mental Health Systems Inc., USA
Deborah Agus
Arden Road, Baltimore, USA
Fred Osher
University of Maryland School of Medicine, USA
David Brown
Baltimore Crisis Response Inc., USA

THE CITY OF BALTIMORE, USA

Baltimore City is the 13th largest city in the United States. It is located on the eastern seaboard of the United States in the state of Maryland 37 miles from Washington, DC and 196 miles from New York City. Baltimore is one of the oldest cities in the USA and in 1997 celebrated the bicentennial of its incorporation. The city is governed by a Mayor and a 19 member City Council which is elected every 4 years.

Over the past 40 years, similar to other urban areas in the USA, Baltimore has experienced a decline in population. Once the largest political jurisdiction in the state of Maryland, with 939,024 or 25% of the state's population, Baltimore is currently the fourth largest subdivision in the state with a population of 692,800 or 14% of the state's population. The majority of the individuals residing in Baltimore City are African-American (about 60%) with Caucasians making up 38% and other races the additional 2%. Baltimore's 14,652 businesses employ 311,161 workers. Manufacturing accounts for 10% of the city's workforce and the largest employer is the Johns Hopkins University and Hospital System.

Indicators of poverty

Baltimore is home to the largest concentration of poor people in Maryland. About one-half of the state's poor people reside in the city of

Baltimore. The population of Baltimore City is about 30% of the metropolitan area (the city and the five surrounding counties) but the city is home to almost 68% of the region's poor. In 1960, the median income of city families was 91.2% of the metropolitan area median family income while in 1990 the income of city families was 66.9% in proportion. (Schmoke & Graves, 1997, p. 15). The poor are overwhelmingly children from single parent homes, African-American female single parents, and the elderly and disabled. (Schmoke & Graves, 1997, p. 16). In 1992, 21.5% of the households in the city had incomes below $10,000 compared to only 9% of households in the state of Maryland. The elderly (over 65 years old) make up 13.7% of the city's population. Over 40% of the elderly population living in the city are disabled, while 32.5% of the elderly state-wide are disabled.

In 1991, the city's unemployment rate of 9.4% was the highest in the state. Baltimore is also home to the greatest concentration of homeless persons and individuals in need of substance abuse treatment in the state.

Baltimore is home to the largest number of Medical Assistance (MA) recipients of any part of Maryland. Eligibility for MA is determined by an individual qualifying for one of several entitlement programmes for poor and/or disabled individuals. The two most frequent entitlement programmes are the Temporary Cash Assistance (TCA) or the Supplemental Security Income (SSI) programme. TCA is for single mothers and their children while the SSI programme is primarily for disabled adults who have not worked enough to qualify for federal programmes such as Social Security or Social Security Disability Income (SSDI). In 1995 there were 187,346 Baltimore residents on the Medicaid programme, which is 27% of the city's population and 40% of the number of MA enrolees state-wide.

MENTAL HEALTH SERVICES IN BALTIMORE

Baltimore Mental Health Systems (BMHS) was created by the Baltimore City Health Department (BCHD) in 1986, and serves as the local mental health authority for Baltimore. In fulfilling its mission to develop a co-ordinated network of care for adults who have serious and persistent mental illnesses and children with serious emotional disturbances, BMHS faced a number of governance and policy issues.

Public mental health services for Baltimore residents are funded by various sources. The two primary sources are Medicaid dollars and State general funds administered by the Mental Hygiene Administration. In the year ending 30 June, 1997, BMHS managed $32 million in state and federal grants that funded a range of out-patient services which generated an additional $20 million in fees through billing Medicaid, Medicare (a federal insurance programme for the elderly and disabled), insurance companies, and client payments. Last year, the system provided out-patient services to 16,282 individuals. The demographics of the individuals receiving services are: 63% African–American, 30% Caucasians, with the majority of the rest Asian or Hispanic individuals; 53% of the individuals are male. Over 50% of the individuals have a major mental illness that includes a diagnosis of schizophrenic disorder, major affective disorder, or other psychotic disorder. About 65% of the individuals live with family members or other unrelated individuals. An estimated 60% of the individuals with a major mental illness have experienced multiple hospitalisations, usually in a state hospital, while an estimated 10% have been incarcerated one or more times for minor offences. Two out of three persons hospitalised in a state hospital are male. About 85% of the individuals with a major mental illness receive Medicaid for health insurance and receive SSI or SSDI as an income entitlement due to their disability (Agus, Blum, & Baron, 1995).

Creation of the local Mental Health Authority

Prior to 1988, the Baltimore City Health Department (BCHD) had responsibility for contracting for mental health services within the city's seven catchment areas (geographic service area). Within each catchment area mental health services were provided by a variety of programmes including community mental health clinics, community rehabilitation programmes (psycho-social) and residential programmes. In addition, several of the areas had emergency room services, and mobile treatment programmes. Although there was a commitment to providing services to individuals with serious mental illness, the services were mostly office-based and often the community relinquished its responsibility for clinical care when an individual refused to keep an appointment, was hospitalised, incarcerated, or became homeless. Services were fragmented and driven by programmatic and fiscal considerations rather than clients' needs. Further, there was no rationale for service development. Instead, historical determinism punctuated by crisis activated decisions and dictated policy. It was a perfect example of a non-system, as described by Stein, Diamond and Factor (1990, p. 213):

> a 'non-system' of mental health care, where a few patients get more than they need, many patients get less than they need, and some get nothing at all. Patients may get lost in this non-system, and no one feels obligated to look for them. Patients may refuse to follow a program's rules and be terminated from treatment by staff who believe that they had no other choice. Patients are moved from the community into the hospital and from the hospital back into the community such that the hospital, the community, the patient, and

the family all feel mistreated. A major problem with this non-system is that it is episode-oriented rather than oriented to provide continuous care.

The purpose of the 'Robert Wood Johnson Foundation (RWJ) Program on Chronic Mental Illness' grant to Baltimore City in 1986 was to enable Baltimore along with eight other large urban areas to develop a coordinated system of care for individuals with serious and persistent mental illnesses. RWJ is the largest health care private foundation in the USA and this project was its first large scale mental health initiative. The city's application to RWJ articulated a need for a local mental health authority to develop a coordinated and comprehensive network of services responsive to the needs of the clients. The city's proposal stated that it would establish a local mental health authority with administrative, clinical, and fiscal authority for the adult mental health system.

The authority would be a public non-profit entity, outside of government, while still maintaining an accountability to government. It would be responsible for coordinating services to create a comprehensive network of community-based care. The authority would focus on expanding the range of services, improving continuity of care, developing new affordable housing opportunities, creating new financing initiatives, and promoting community acceptance and public education.

Upon receiving the grant, the City established BMHS as the local mental health authority for Baltimore City. It operates through a Board of Directors comprising government officials, community leaders, and primary and secondary consumers of mental health services. BMHS has been responsible for distributing funds to servicc providers, re-designing the structure for the system of delivering and financing services, creating new services, monitoring quality of care, promoting continuity of care, establishing a computerised Client Information System, and developing affordable housing. BMHS envisions a coordinated network of services controlled by a strong, centralised local mental health authority which is responsive and accountable to the varying demands of the individuals it serves. Within this mandate the goals of BMHS are to:

1. Provide quality care.
2. Ensure continuity of care.
3. Use scarce resources efficiently.

Over the past 10 years, BMHS has made major strides in accomplishing these goals. BMHS has:

1. Redesigned the delivery system by consolidating providers into Lead Agencies.

2. Expanded the range of services to include mobile outreach, and services to homeless individuals with mental illness.
3. Increased case management services.
4. Increased linkages between state hospitals and out-patient providers to improve continuity of care.
5. Created affordable housing through its non-profit housing development corporation, Community Housing Associates, Inc.
6. Established Baltimore Crisis Response, Inc. to coordinate and provide a full range of crisis services.
7. Established an employment training program for primary consumers to be employed within the mental health system.
8. Developed a major capitated financing demonstration to better integrate fiscal incentives with good care.

CHOICES IN CREATING A LOCAL MENTAL HEALTH AUTHORITY

Many of the decisions made in determining the design to be used in Baltimore are fundamental to creating a service delivery system anywhere. The difference in local condition might affect the ultimate decision, but the issues and choices are universal. The following describes several of these broad issues, the rationale for choosing a particular design option, and the impact of that design on system of care in Baltimore.

Whether to provide any direct services

Authorities or regulators face this dilemma: Is it best to control services by providing them, by having others provide them, or by a combination of the above?

The mixed role, of regulator and provider, presents certain advantages. First, there is greater control both in terms of defining a service and fitting it into a cohesive, clinical network. Second, it is easier to coordinate, to provide consistency and to adapt more quickly a particular service to needs. By combining the management and policy setting roles with direct service, one enjoys a stronger linkage and, maybe, a quicker response time between systemic needs and priorities, and the services provided.

BMHS nonetheless chose not to be a direct service provider for the following reasons. First, if one is both a provider and a regulator/payer there is a confusion of roles with a strong potential for conflict of interest in areas of quality assurance, redefinition of services, and allocation of new funds for services (Stein et al., 1990, p. 216).

Second, as a competitor with other providers, yet with authority for managing the system, there might be a perception of inequality or favouritism, causing the decisions of BMHS to be viewed suspiciously or sceptically. BMHS would have difficulty acting as an arbiter and manager, as an authority, when instead of being above the fray it was in the middle of it. Therefore, BMHS determined that it was unwise to compromise itself by providing services.

Although this issue was resolved early in the development of BMHS, it has arisen again from time to time as new services develop, and the temptation to take a more active role persists. For example, after investing much time and resources on developing a model for a new crisis system, there was some feeling that the new centralised crisis centre should be under the direct control of BMHS. Members of BMHS board of directors felt it was 'their baby' and that they should ensure that it fulfilled its promise and adhered to specific principles by directly operating the service. However, although the new role was enticing, after re-examining the original rationale for avoiding direct services, the BMHS board reaffirmed its role and established an independent crisis system provider which BMHS monitors through its contract with the provider. Understanding why one is making a decision and examining the short and long-term ramifications within a framework, clarifies the issue and facilitates reasoned decision-making.

Centralisation *vs* decentralisation of services

Baltimore City, as noted earlier, is divided into seven catchment areas each of which had an existing array of services when BMHS started. BMHS considered options ranging from the one extreme of centralising all services, to the other of centralising no services and having a multitude of separate providers for each service. The middle ground options, were to have either the regional services or to centralise only certain specialised services.

BMHS decided that the core services should exist in each area but should be consolidated under the auspices of one strong area authority: the Lead Agency. Decisions on specialised services would be made on a case by case basis. Consolidating the providers under the Lead Agency umbrella reflects both the desire to emphasise the comprehensive needs of individual clients rather than strengthening individual programmes into which clients then need to fit, and the desire to create a strong constituency at the direct service, or local level. Theoretically, we have retained the strong neighbourhood affiliation and enhanced the accountability of the providers by combining them within a Lead Agency whose mission is to serve all clients, and all needs, regardless of affiliation with a specific provider/programme or lack thereof. Each Lead Agency is then a part of the larger coordinated system of care under the aegis of BMHS.

Thus, at the direct service level, services are decentralised by being controlled and consolidated at the local level within the Lead Agency, while decisions on planning, management and funding are centralised under BMHS. As new specialised services are developed, BMHS analyses the benefits of centralising or decentralising that service, balancing systemic needs with the role of the Lead Agencies and neighbourhood needs. For example, in the realm of services to homeless persons, a recent discussion centred on the issue of whether to create a specialised city-wide provider for mental health services to homeless persons, or to continue to encourage/require the Lead Agencies to reach out and integrate homeless individuals into their programmes.

The benefits of centralisation relate to control, speed, and direction: one provider with a clearly defined mission can act more quickly and definitively to serve its specifically targeted population. Additionally, since people who are 'homeless' by definition do not actually reside in a catchment area, it was argued that services should not be catchment area based. The benefits of decentralisation are those of long-term integration, accountability of Lead Agencies for comprehensive services and the best use of available resources for the entire system within which homeless services are a part. BMHS believes that people who are homeless and mentally ill resemble the majority of the target population for out-patient services once they are housed: homelessness is at times a consequence of the mental illness and in any event is not, and should not be treated as, a permanent condition. Using the framework of the Lead Agency system as a focal point for decision-making, and applying and examining the benefits, and concomitant disadvantages, described above, BMHS determined that homeless services should remain with the Lead Agencies. Attention has focused on strengthening the Lead Agencies' commitment to, and accountability for, this population without creating a new, separate, service. This decision is opposite to that made for crisis services where different elements, e.g. the acute and specialised nature of the services, prevailed, outweighing the arguments for decentralisation. Similarly, in providing services to children and adolescents, we have determined that the best approach to delivering services to children and adolescents who have complex problems is the establishment of a city-wide service.

Division of power: intrusive *vs* guided management

A central authority with clearly articulated goals, and without direct-service responsibility, must determine whether the best way to achieve these goals is through direct intervention in the interstices of a service provider's business or by macro-management through specified goals and outcome criteria. These options are easily understood with reference to the clinical or financial arena. For example, a mental health authority has the option either to monitor and approve a very specific budget and all modifications thereto, or to allow budget flexibility as long as the outcome criteria, such as improved client functioning in vocational areas, are met. Similarly, the authority might choose either to mandate specific numbers of units of services which must be provided to each client, or instead use an outcome measure such as quality of life indicators. There is of course, as in each decision, a full spectrum of alternatives from which the authority might choose, and additionally it can mix and match, i.e. flexibility in clinical issues but strict controls in financial areas. There are also limitations to flexibility imposed by external factors such as state law, and by internal factors such as the ability of the authority to perform quality assurance reviews measuring subtle indicators.

BMHS is taking an evolutionary approach: the goal is towards increased flexibility but the reality is that we are reaching this incrementally as we educate ourselves, our providers, and the state. In spite of its commitment to this principle, day-to-day issues tempt BMHS with micro-management and we struggle to sort out which decisions to make and how involved we should be. Flexibility is risky but the potential benefits of greater creativity and empowerment of consumers and providers to respond to individual needs, justifies the risk. Other authorities might determine that the safety of greater control outweighs the risk in their system.

The capitation demonstration developed by BMHS and supported by the state, and described in detail later in this paper, is designed to explore fully the potential of 'guided management'. The demonstration allows a good deal of flexibility and autonomy at the Lead Agency level in exchange for stringent quality assurance and articulated outcome criteria contained in a negotiated contract.

SYSTEM REDESIGN: LEAD AGENCY

One of the first tasks of BMHS was redesigning the service delivery system to create Lead Agencies. BMHS organised individual service providers in each catchment area into a Lead Agency, whose overall mission is to reach out to persons in their area with chronic mental illness regardless of whether they are a client of any one of the existing programmes. The design has been built on the principle that providers as a group must shed their programmatic territorialism and consider the 'whole' client rather than pigeonholing clients within programmatic barriers.

Each Lead Agency is headed either by the Chairman of the Department of Psychiatry, in the five hospital-based agencies, or by the Executive Director of the free-standing corporation in the remaining two areas. There is a Lead Agency governing consortium comprised of the heads of each service component. Contracts between BMHS and the Lead Agency describe the structure of the Agency and delineate both the Lead Agencies' and BMHS's responsibilities. Therefore at the provider level, services are decentralised, controlled at the community level, and consolidated within one local agency. However, decisions on planning, priorities, management, and funding are centralised under the aegis of BMHS.

The Lead Agencies grapple with issues of coordinating care and respond to clinical and planning issues raised by BMHS. The Lead Agency directors meet as a group with the President of BMHS to discuss system-wide issues and concerns. It is BMHS's expectation that local input, derived from client-centred service providers, will drive the planning of future systems.

This network of care reflects an 'adaptation to local conditions', such as the pre-existing neighbourhood-based catchment area system and the presence of several large general hospitals with hospital-based community psychiatry programmes. One such hospital is the University of Maryland Medical Systems (UMMS), whose Department of Psychiatry was designated as a Lead Agency in 1993.

UMMS provides mental health services to the 160,000 residents of south and southwest Baltimore. In this capacity, the UMMS Lead Agency develops, provides, and evaluates community mental health services to persons with serious mental illnesses and children with serious emotional disturbances. The Department of Psychiatry has a long history of academic excellence and commitment to community services and has emphasised state-of-the-art administrative and community-based services. Of the more than 1900 active adult patients served by the UMMS Lead Agency last year, more than 40% (790 patients) have a diagnosis of schizophrenia. Services within the UMMS Lead Agency closely parallel the ideal community support system described by the Community Support Program of National Institute of Mental Health (NIMH) (Stroul, 1984). They include out-patient mental health and addiction services, psychosocial rehabilitation, vocational services, housing, entitlements, crisis response services, and assertive community treatment. Consumer and family involvement are strongly supported. These programmes make up a continuum of care critical to successful outcomes for persons with severe mental illnesses.

The UMMS Lead Agency has a continuum of treatment services with three levels of care. Approximately 20% of the individuals with Serious and Persistent Mental Illness (SPMI) receive services in specialised high intensity teams modelled closely after the Program in Assertive Community Treatment (PACT Team) programme. The PACT clients typically have had multiple psychiatric hospitalisations and high use of emergency room services with poor out-patient compliance. Non-medical PACT staff (social workers, case managers, consumer staff) have a caseload of approximately 12 clients, and the staff:patient ratio for PACT psychiatrists is 1:75. The UMMS PACT team has a specific mission to include homeless adults with severe mental illnesses in Baltimore and includes consumer advocates to facilitate outreach and engagement of this disaffiliated subgroup. These consumer advocates are paid staff members who have a history of homelessness and/or mental illness. They do not carry a caseload, but assist patients in meeting their treatment goals. They are often instrumental in engaging patients and in locating patients who drop out of contact, provide peer counselling, and serve as role models for patients.

An additional 20% of Lead Agency patients are served in a mid-level intensity team with higher consumer/staff ratios but which still embraces many key PACT elements (Continuous Care Team (CCT)). Non-medical CCT staff have a caseload of approximately 25 clients, and the staff: patient ratio for CCT psychiatrists is 1:100. In the UMMS Lead Agency the two speciality teams, PACT and CCT, differ in ways outlined below, yet each provides mobile, interdisciplinary, comprehensive, 24-hour, continuous (in-patient/out-patient) care with a one-stop shop approach. In addition, the teams employ a full-time family outreach worker who is a family member of a consumer. These workers participate with the teams in treatment planning and provide support and education for family members. They assist with the planning and conducting of family meetings and run family group interventions as described by McFarlane, Lukens, Lint, Dushay, Deakins, Newmark, Dunne, Horen, and Toray (1995). Sixty-five percent of the individuals served have a diagnosis of a schizophrenic disorder.

The remaining 60% of the SPMI population is served within two out-patient clinics with adjunctive case management available. The non-medical therapists in the clinics have case ratios of 1:65 while a full-time psychiatrist has a caseload of 1:200. Very little off-site care is provided and when hospitalisation is necessary, care is coordinated via phone contact between in-patient and community providers.

Because of the high prevalence of persons with co-occurring addictive and mental disorders, each team and clinic provides integrated substance abuse treatment services with individual and group interventions. Crisis services for individuals receiving care within the Lead Agency are provided by the speciality teams through on-call coverage, while patients served in the out-patient clinics can receive immediate, 24-hour response and intervention to crises within a hospital-based psychiatric urgent care system. This includes the capacity for brief intensive care management until the person can be engaged in other Lead Agency programmes in the city. The Lead Agency has a close working relationship with Baltimore Crisis Response, Inc. (BCRI) which provides crisis services for individuals in need of mobile crisis and crisis residential services.

Assignment of a patient to a level of care is based upon the client's score on the Multnomah Community Assessment Scale, the Substance Abuse Treatment Scale (SATS), and clinical judgement. The CAS is a 17–item instrument designed to be completed by case managers and gives a measure of the patient's severity of disability. It was originally developed for persons with chronic and severe mental illnesses and is administered at the UMMS Lead Agency programmes during baseline evaluation and every three months thereafter. This instrument is used to rate the client on ability to structure daily activities, social effectiveness, treatment compliance, frequency of crises and other dimensions which assist in determining the intensity of out-patient treatment needed as well as providing outcome data on key dimensions. The UMMS Lead Agency has modified the Alcohol/Drug Abuse item on the CAS to be the five-point clinician alcohol/drug use scale (CRS) developed by Drake, Osher, and Wallach (1989). The CRS corresponds to DSM–III–R criteria, has been shown to be reliable, sensitive, and specific when used by case managers, and does not change the overall CAS score. Patients scoring between 20–50 on the CAS are typically assigned to the PACT team, between 35–65 to the CCT, and between 50–80 to the out-patient clinics. The SATS (McHugo, Drake, Burton, & Ackerson, 1995), used with persons who are dually diagnosed, combines a motivational hierarchy with explicit substance use criteria to form an eight-stage scale of the recovery process. The SATS is used as both an assessment instrument and outcome measure. The UMMS Lead Agency provides ongoing training to case managers on the use of these measures. Referrals to level of care go through a single evaluator and monthly meetings of all Lead Agency medical and programme directors address case assignment issues. For services not directly provided within the UMMS Lead Agency (i.e. in-patient care at the Carter Center, a state operated acute in-patient care facility, supported employment at the Schapiro Training and Employment Program, a city-wide supported employment programme, and BCRI), interagency agreements have been developed.

EXPANDING AND CREATING SERVICES IN RESPONSE TO SYSTEM-WIDE NEED

This focus on systemic issues did not prevent BMHS from concomitantly expanding and restructuring services. To the contrary, consistent with the principles enunciated above, BMHS has developed services, and programmes, as described below, which have had a profound impact on the treatment of individuals with severe and persistent mental illness.

Expansion of the range of services

For the past 10 years, BMHS has focused on increasing mobile services particularly to individuals not well served by the mental health system. BMHS has established a Case Management Unit (CMU) within each Lead Agency and has provided resources to allow each CMU to hire staff to provide intensive, brokering case management services. There have been over 30 new case management positions created along with the development of the State of Maryland's first Medicaid funded mental health case management programme. Through these resources the mental health system has assumed responsibility for individuals who fail to keep appointments and who reject traditional mental health services. The following vignette describes an individual who is typical of many of the individuals receiving case management services:

> Mr. C is a 39-year-old male with chronic undifferentiated schizophrenia. Since the age of 8, Mr. C has spent most of his life in institutions. Over the past 20 years, his life has been grossly disorganised. He has had numerous arrests for disturbing the peace, urinating in public, loitering, and attempting to direct traffic. Before his involvement with the case management programme, he had not remained in the community longer than five consecutive months. He was almost always homeless, had extremely poor hygiene, and wore unseasonal clothes.
>
> Mr. C was assigned a case manager and his case manager began working with him on what would prove to be a long and challenging endeavour toward keeping him out of the hospital and engaged in out-patient treatment. Initially, his case manager accompanied Mr. C to all appointments while working to develop a rapport based on support and mutual trust. Eventually she discontinued escorting him to the clinic and began calling transportation for him, each time phoning both the client and the bus services more than once to ensure follow-through. After a couple of months of having transportation arranged for him, he began to use the phone to call transportation himself. Slowly, he learned how to call for appointments and even to reschedule missed appointments.
>
> The past year has brought many positive changes for Mr. C. He was fitted for dentures. He paid back in full a BMHS loan which was provided for his dental care. Mr. C connected with his family, and together they have moved into a brand new fully furnished three bedroom apartment with central heat and air, washer and dryer, and dishwasher available through BMHS's housing subsidiary Community Housing Associates (CHA). He is currently paying on his second BMHS loan approved for the payment of the security deposit on his new home. He reports living the life he has wanted for many years but needed support and encouragement to attain.

BMHS has prioritised expanding services to individuals who have a serious mental illness and are homeless. Through BMHS's efforts, services to the homeless mentally ill have been expanded in Lead Agencies in five of the city's seven catchment areas. In addition, BMHS was a successful applicant for a three year, three million dollar NIMH grant which established the assertive community treatment team at UMMS, has been a partner in the Office of Homeless Services successful federal applications that has created assertive community treatment teams for two additional Lead Agencies, and has been a co-sponsor with the local and state housing authority for grants to support affordable housing for homeless mentally ill individuals.

Crisis care

The backbone of a good community-based mental health system is the presence of an emergency system which is comprehensive, well coordinated, and committed to providing a range of community alternatives (Stein et al., 1990, p. 213) In its role as the manager of the system, BMHS convened a task force that met for a year and developed a plan to redesign the psychiatric crisis system. The report called for the creation of a new entity to operate mobile crisis services, to manage crisis residential alternatives, to provide information and referral services, to have authority over pre-admission screening, and to coordinate the emergency services provided by the emergency rooms and community mental health clinics of the Lead Agencies. This plan established Baltimore Crisis Response Inc (BCRI).

BCRI is a community-based crisis intervention programme. The mission of the agency is to assist adults experiencing mental health crises by providing timely, effective, crisis services in the most therapeutic and least restrictive environment possible. Specifically, the goal is to treat people in the community and prevent unnecessary in-patient admissions to psychiatric hospitals. BCRI, which began operating in May, 1993, provides three clinical services to the community. These services are:

1. Information, Referral, Crisis Hotline: The hotline is available to the metropolitan Baltimore area and operates 24 hours a day, seven days a week. The hotline provides crisis counselling, suicide prevention, and community referrals. The hotline operates as the gateway to the Mobile Crisis Team and receives about 10,000 calls annually.
2. Mobile Crisis Team: The Mobile Crisis Team (MCT) (including a psychiatrist, nurse, mental health counsellor and case associate) is dispatched in Baltimore City. The team operates from 8am-11pm, responds to people in crisis in their homes, shelters, hospitals, and other community locations. The MCT assesses the person in crisis,

initiates interventions (crisis counselling, starts medications), and makes linkages to mental health services and other community resources. A psychiatrist and mental health professional are available 24 hours a day, 7 days a week.

3. Crisis Residential Alternatives: The crisis residential intervention includes in-home support or crisis beds and operates as an alternative to in-patient hospitalisation. In the event that the person needs additional support in home, BCRI can provide in-home mental health counsellors. The counsellors can stay in the person's home up to 48 hours, assist in transporting the person to appointments, monitor medications and provide emotional and behavioural support. This service can be provided for 48 hours around the clock or in increments (i.e. for 5 hours a day up to 8 days). If the person does not have a supportive home environment, BCRI also operates crisis beds. The crisis beds are supervised 24 hours a day. Services include daily counselling, medication monitoring, linkages to community services, and daily transportation to health and mental health appointments for up to 5 days. The goal is for the person to be clinically stabilised and linked to appropriate community resources prior to discharge.

Improvements in continuity of care

The community frequently relinquishes its responsibility for clinical care when an individual is hospitalised, incarcerated, or becomes homeless. BMHS's Lead Agency agreements require each Lead Agency to assume responsibility for individuals regardless of where they are living. BMHS also established a project to improve continuity of care for individuals being discharged from State Hospitals known as the Service Area Co-ordinator initiative. The project has as its central concept the designation of responsibility to a Lead Agency for each patient being discharged from a state hospital. BMHS staff are responsible for linking patients to Lead Agencies by referring them to the Case Management Unit of the appropriate Lead Agency. This process not only improves continuity of care, it encourages the hospital and community to work together with the patient to create an individualised plan for community living.

Case managers from the Lead Agency are charged in all cases with the responsibility of developing and carrying through an individualised plan for the patient's return to the community. The Lead Agencies depend on their Case Management Units (CMU) to provide services to individuals wherever the persons may be living. It has not been unusual for the CMU staff to work with a client six months prior to his leaving the state hospital, or to develop housing opportunities for an individual whom they met in a homeless shelter.

An important element of continuity of care is the availability of information which allows for client tracking and system utilisation reviews. BMHS has developed a Client Information System (CIS) based on a unique identifier which compiles demographic and utilisation information on individuals seen in the public out-patient system and discharged from a state hospital. The CIS has developed reports which identify multiple users of emergency rooms and state hospitals who have not been seen by the community mental health clinics. Attempts have been made to target these individuals for intensive case management services.

Creation of community housing associates to develop housing

Community Housing Associates, Inc. (CHA) is a non-profit organisation whose primary mission is the development of affordable housing in Baltimore City for persons with mental illness. CHA is a subsidiary of Baltimore Mental Health Systems, Inc. (BMHS), and was established in 1989. Through its close relationship with BMHS, CHA ensures that tenants have access to mental health services.

CHA has developed 400 units of housing for persons with mental illness through a variety of funding strategies, which include use of State loan and grants, federal government assistance, funds from the Robert Wood Johnson Foundation and federal tax credits. Also CHA manages 200 Section 8 certificates and 190 Shelter Plus Care sponsor-based rental assistance beds. Section 8 is a federal programme that provides housing assistance to poor individuals in which the tenant only pays about 30% of their income towards rent. Shelter Plus Care is another federal programme and closely resembles Section 8 except that it is restricted to disabled individuals who are homeless. Some of the rental subsidies are used to operate CHA-owned housing and the rest are used to lease units from private owners. CHA's housing activities are coordinated with BMHS-funded mental health providers and tenants are able to access housing in any area of Baltimore City.

Access to CHA housing is limited to low-income people who have a history of mental illness. There is no requirement for participation in programmes or services as tenants sign a lease and the only way they can lose their housing is if they choose to move elsewhere or break their lease.

Development of capitation demonstration project integrating clinical and fiscal structures

People with schizophrenia and other major mental illnesses require a comprehensive, diverse and ever-changing range of services over a long period of time. Moreover, because of the complex and chronic, yet episodic, nature of the disease, each client presents different needs over time. However, traditional financing is fragmented, relatively inflexible, and programme specific. Furthermore, the incentives created by current financing often encourage providers to use less than optimal approaches to treatment. BMHS developed a planning process using a Capitation Work Group comprised of mental health financing specialists, and a representative from the state Mental Hygiene Administration and the State Medicaid Agency, which established the Capitation Demonstration Proposal to address this problem. Implementation of the Project started in the autumn of 1994 with the hiring of staff and training and the first client enrolled in May 1995.

The purpose of the demonstration is to reconfigure the financing system to facilitate high quality, comprehensive care to clients in the community with individualised, flexible and innovative treatment plans. Specific goals are:

1. To increase the accessibility of services to those who often face barriers.
2. To increase the continuum of services, including services that are useful but not easily paid for under current funding.
3. To reduce the use of expensive general hospital bed days and enrich community services accordingly.
4. To develop fiscal integrity for the local system and increase ability to plan for the future.
5. To provide predictable costs for funders while encouraging creative and entrepreneurial activity, with retention of savings in carry-over funds.

The design of the Project is as follows:

1. There will be 300 clients enrolled in one of two capitation Lead Agencies. The Lead Agencies were chosen pursuant to a competitive Request for Proposals open to all seven Lead Agencies.
2. The 300 clients will be persons who are diagnosed with a severe and persistent mental illness and who are currently in a state hospital or who have been discharged from a state or general hospital within the past two years. At least one-third will be current state hospital residents who have been hospitalised for at least six months.

3. The state transfers to BMHS a lump sum payment comprised of Medicaid dollars and state grant dollars previously used to fund state hospitals and community services.
4. BMHS takes money off the top for administration purposes (3.5% of rate) and to place into an incentive account (1.5%) and a risk pool (2.0%).
5. BMHS then pays, quarterly, the remainder of the capitated rate to the Lead Agency multiplied by the number of enrolees.
6. With this payment, the Lead Agencies are required, by contract, to pay for all of the enrolee's mental health needs including in-patient hospitalisation. They are also required to provide for meeting other needs such as health, dental, housing and substance abuse treatment and are allowed to use capitation funds for these purposes as necessary. They are also allowed to use these funds in other creative ways to pay for items or services that are non-traditional but necessary for the client's success.
7. BMHS monitors services throughout the year using threshold criteria and face to face meetings, and then contracts for an annual independent evaluation.
8. The CLAs are evaluated according to outcome criteria reflecting a client's quality of life. These outcome criteria include positive indicators such as employment and independent housing, as well as systems indicators such as hospitalisation and jail time which BMHS wants to reduce.
9. Pursuant to the evaluation, each Agency receives a grade which determines whether the Agency will receive funds from the incentive account and whether they will be able to retain up to 85% of their unspent funds. Thus, monetary incentives are directly related to quality of care.
10. The unspent funds returned to BMHS are apportioned between the Risk Pool and a Development Account for new services thus spreading risk and savings across the system.
11. Finally, and most importantly, BMHS is responsible for providing leadership and vision and translating that into action through an ongoing training programme.

After three years, there are 163 clients currently enrolled, 120 of whom had been in a state hospital at least six months in their last stay. The average length of last stay is seven years. The following story illustrates the benefits of the Project.

Mr. Brown was hospitalised for nine continuous years before leaving Springfield State Hospital, a Maryland State Hospital, in June, 1994. His goals were

> 'to find a job, open a bank account, and to have my own apartment'. Mr. Brown has been working 20 hours per week in a second-hand store for three years. He is presently looking for a full-time job. He enjoys buying clothes and items for his apartment with the money he saves from each paycheck. This September, Mr. Brown plans to renew his apartment lease for the third year. According to his sister, 'We were told by doctors in the hospital that my brother couldn't live in the community. Now he has his own apartment, he's got a job. We're so proud of him.'

Like the benefits, the challenges involved in implementing this Project are numerous. First, the clients have exhibited a very high degree of serious, physical illness resulting in a higher than expected mortality rate (11 deaths) and a great deal of time and effort spent in improving linkages to health care. Second, when greater flexibility and risk-taking are encouraged, it is constantly necessary to balance reasonable risk with high support and prudent oversight. There are also many issues related to housing such as safety, affordability, cleanliness, client choice and whether to enforce minimum guidelines.

Yet, with all of these challenges, the Project has been quite successful. Both programmes have created teams with social workers, nurses, psychiatrists and consumers who work together to meet the client's needs. The teams are empowered to use their skills and resources creatively to meet a client's needs. For example, one project has used some funds to create a job at a hospital for its clients by agreeing to pay part of the salary. All staff work at developing unique relationships and challenging themselves and their clients to reach their full potential.

Both programmes received an 'A' minus on last years evaluation while realising substantial savings. Plans are currently underway to use money in BMHS's Development Account for a joint project for job development. There will also be a joint endeavour to create some new resources for persons with mental illness and substance abuse diagnoses.

A unique feature of this model is its combination of mechanical innovations, the financing, and state-of-the art clinical approaches supported by training and by the focus on outcomes related to quality of life. In this project, BMHS has fully realised the concept of guided management by focusing on goals rather than mandating specific services, processes or staffing patterns.

IMPLICATIONS FOR OTHER SYSTEMS

As described above, each decision on an element of management or governance leads to specific decisions on programmatic, fiscal and clinical issues. There are other decisions beyond those analysed above which can only be mentioned briefly, such as whether to restrict the number of providers, as BMHS did, or to encourage many unrelated and competing providers as the new MHA system design is doing. Other decisions will face us in the future and will be determined largely by reference to the initial principles and goals articulated by the framework of the system design.

As mental health authorities develop in other locales, the first task should be to determine values, set overriding goals and then develop the framework to meet these goals based on the general issues described in this paper. Then when specific issues arise they can be addressed coherently within this framework, rather than in an ad hoc, serendipitous manner.

BMHS has articulated the values of a flexible system of high-quality comprehensive services designed to meet the needs of all adults with severe and persistent mental illness and children, adolescents and their families with serious emotional disturbances. The system redesign and service initiatives reflect these values as will future decisions. The focus on long-term structural change rather than dramatic, rapid clinical service change is difficult to maintain but, we firmly believe, worthwhile. The results will be far-reaching, permanent and comprehensive.

THE FUTURE

The funding and organisation of public mental health services in Maryland changed on 1 July 1997. Based on approval from the federal government, the state of Maryland placed the majority of individuals on Medicaid in managed care. Until that time the individual's medical and psychiatric care was not managed and the individual had the choice to see any provider who was authorised by Medicaid to provide the service. In the new system, the recipients will have a medical home within a Managed Care Organisation (MCO). The MCO is responsible for providing all somatic care, including substance abuse treatment, while mental health services are carved out of this system. The Mental Hygiene Administration (MHA), the state mental health authority, was authorised to develop a Speciality Mental Health System. MHA's design has several components. They are:

1. The system has contracted with a behavioural health organisation to serve as an administrative services organisation (ASO).
2. The ASO will manage access to care and utilisation, pay claims, develop data from claims, and conduct evaluation.
3. The system will be primarily fee-for-service and for the first time the mental health system will manage the dollars spent for in-patient care. In 1995 Medicaid spent $84 million on mental health care for

Baltimore City residents of which $49 million or 58% was spent on inpatient care.

BMHS as the Core Service Agency for the city of Baltimore will enter into an agreement with the ASO to manage the system. There are several issues that will emerge in the first few years of the new design. They include:

1. Whether there is a role for BMHS as a strong local mental health authority in the new fee-for-service in which approximately 85% of the dollars will be paid through fee-for-service.
2. Whether BMHS will be able to design initiatives that target the most in need, i.e. an expansion of BMHS's specially designed mental health capitation project for adults and the development of demonstration projects for children and adolescents.
3. Whether BMHS's ability to develop special initiatives and features of its mental health system that may be unique to the city of Baltimore will be supported by the state.

REFERENCES

Agus, D., Blum, S., & Baron, S. (1995). Building a capitated public mental health service for seriously mentally ill adults: The Baltimore experience. *Administration and Policy in Mental Health, 22*, 261–271.

Drake, R.E., Osher, F.C., & Wallach, M.A. (1989). Alcohol use and abuse in schizophrenia: A prospective community study. *Journal of Nervous and Mental Diseases, 177*, 404–414.

McFarlane, W.R., Lukens, E., Link, B., Dushay, R., Deakins, S.A., Newmark, M., Dunne, E.J., Horen, B., & Toran, J. (1995). Multiple-family groups and psychoeducation in the treatment of schizophrenia. *Archives of General Psychiatry, 52*, 679–687.

McHugo, G.J., Drake, R.E., Burton, H.L., & Ackerson, T.M. (1995). A scale for assessing the stage of substance abuse treatment in persons with severe mental illness. *Journal of Nervous and Mental Disease, 183*, 762–767.

Schmoke, K.L., Mayor, Graves, C.C. III, Director. (1997, February). Baltimore: Past, present and future trends and projections. Baltimore: Baltimore City Planning Department.

Stein, L.M.D., Diamond, R.M.D., & Factor, R.M.D. (1990). A system approach to the care of persons with schizophrenia. *Handbook of Schizophrenia, Vol. 5, Psychosocial Therapies* Amsterdam: Elsevier Science.

Stroul, B. (1984). *Toward community support systems for the mentally disabled: The NIMH Community Support Program.* Boston: Center for Psychiatric Rehabilitation, Sargent College of Allied Health Professions.

CHAPTER FIVE

The city of Bangalore, India

R. Srinivasa Murthy
National Institute of Mental Health and Neuro Sciences, Bangalore, India

INTRODUCTION

Jawaharlal Nehru, the first Prime Minister of independent India, named Bangalore 'India's city of the future'. Bangalore is the most Westernised, and the most cosmopolitan Indian city. Bangalore symbolises the emerging India which is progressive and vibrant, and represents a country in transition. Up until about two decades ago Bangalore was known as 'a pensioner's paradise', but it is now more popularly known as the 'silicon valley of India'. It covers an area of 366 km^2 and has a population of 4,807,019 (1991 census). At 920 metres above sea level it has a warm, pleasant climate with an average annual rainfall of 859.6 mm. Kannada, Tamil, Hindi, and English are widely spoken. Its major industries include, aeronautics, telecommunications, electronics, computer engineering, computer software, electrical, machine tools, watch-making, breweries and distilleries, handicrafts, silk processing, garment export, granite and horticulture.

THE CITY OF BANGALORE

History

27 BC	Coins of Roman emperors found at Yeswanthpur.
850 AD	The name Bangalore occurs for the first time on a 9th century stone inscription.

1024	Part of Chola empire.
1537	Kempegowda builds the town.
1638	Conquered by the Bijapur Army.
1640–44	Maratha rule.
1687	Moghul rule.
1799	Wodeyar family of Mysore kingdom.
1809	British cantonment.
1831–81	British rule.
1881	Maharaja's rule.
1937	Mental Hospital, Bangalore.
1949	Bangalore Municipal corporation.
1955	Modern state legislature (Vidhana Soudha) built.
1956	Capital of unified greater Mysore.
1961–71	Industrial townships of aeronautics, telecommunications, machine tools, watches, electrical equipment.
1980	Preferred location of computer hardware and software companies.

Independence brought radical changes in Mysore state. Mysore state became an integral part of India politically, with the Maharaja losing his powers and making way for an elected government. The capital of the state was shifted from Mysore to Bangalore in 1956 (Gazettes of India, 1990).

Bangalore is unusual among the Indian cities in that it is a centre for both hi-tech industries and advanced research in the sciences and technology. This happy mix of industry and research is a factor in its recent emergence as a world-class centre for computer software design, and also a centre for foreign investment.

Area

In 1961, there was a sudden and substantial increase in the area of Bangalore city. During the last three decades a number of new areas have been added, to resulting in the current size of the city. The density of population in 1901 was 5624 per km^2, but it had doubled by 1991. The current density of population, 11,196 per km^2, is less than that for other major cities of India.

Population

Bangalore emerged as a million population city during the decade of 1951–61. Currently Bangalore is the fifth largest city in India. The population growth of Bangalore city as well as of its urban agglomeration was uneven: slow up to 1941, then an unprecedented growth rate of 91% was observed between 1941 and 1951. During 1971–81, the city experienced its second boom of population growth measuring about a 75% increase. The population is doubling every 20 years, and in 1991 was 4.09 million for greater Bangalore, and 3.26 million for the city. One of the major contributors to growth of population is migration. It is estimated that 110,000 of the population are life-time migrants, up to 1981 forming about 37% of the total population. Of the total migrants, 54% of the migrants came to the city during the 1971–81 period. Economic factors related to employment and/or family migration was the reason in 59% of cases.

Age groups

Table 5.1 presents the age distribution of the population for males and females.

The sex ratio shows that there is a predominance of male population. In 1901, the sex ratio of Bangalore was 961 females for 1000 males; and in 1991 it was 909 in 1991. This ratio is better than for many cities of India, for example Bombay (819), Calcutta (827), and Delhi (831).

Marital status

It is estimated that 60% of males and 50% of females are never married. The proportion of never married females in the age group of 15–34 has shown a sharp rise in 1981 as compared to 1971 (33% *vs* 20%). It is also found that the proportion of widowed/separated/divorced women is as high as 50% for females in the age group of 50+ years, as compared to only 10% for males. This could be a reflection of the remarriage of men, while females remain widowed.

TABLE 5.1
Percentage Distribution of Population by Age and Sex during 1971 and 1981

Age	*Males*		*Females*		*Total*	
	1971	1981	1971	1981	1971	1981
<15	35.74	33.73	39.89	36.87	37.67	35.22
15–19	10.45	10.25	10.78	10.78	10.60	10.50
20–29	20.65	21.05	20.26	21.15	20.45	1.09
30–39	14.09	14.70	12.48	12.90	13.34	13.85
40–49	9.50	9.75	7.54	7.80	8.59	8.89
50–59	5.22	5.43	4.56	5.02	4.92	5.23
60+	4.35	5.05	4.49	5.48	4.43	5.26

TABLE 5.2
The Literacy Rate for Bangalore, 1961–1991

Year	*Males*	*Females*	*Total*
1961	59.68	39.12	50.06
1971	65.68	51.27	58.95
1981	70.26	57.75	64.36
1991*	73.74	62.86	68.95

* Children in the age group 0–6 are not considered in the numerator for calculating literacy rate.

Literacy

The literacy rate is increasing with time, and is greater for males than females (see Table 5.2) (Bhattacharjee & Yadav, 1993).

Religion

The religious composition of the city consists of six major religious groups—namely Hindus (78%), Muslims (14%), Christians (7%), Jains (1%), Sikhs (0.09%), and Buddhists (0.01%). The growth rates of the different religious groups is about the same as the decadal growth rate of the city population.

Language

The major languages spoken by the population are Kannada (34%), Tamil (23%), Telugu (16%), Urdu (14%), Malayalam (3%), Marathi (3%), and Hindi (2%).

Occupation

The overall proportion categorised as workers is 33%. There is a great disparity between the males (83%) and females (18%) in the total working population (1991 data). There has recently been an increase in women in the working group, from 13.3% in 1981 to current levels. The major occupational groups are in the industries and manufacturing followed by other services and trade.

Public Amenities

The Population Crisis Committee, Washington (1990) report on the top 100 metropolitan cities of the world includes nine Indian cities, including

Bangalore, and rates the indicators of living standard as 'poor' in all the nine cities. Bangalore is not located next to a major river. Until 1896, the city was supplied water without any purification treatment. The first water supply scheme was planned at the turn of the century for a population of 0.25 million. The next major development was to bring water from the Arkavathy river about 40 km from Bangalore. The additional major source of water to the city is from the River Cauvery which is over 100 km from the city.

In recent years there has been a perpetual shortage of power. As against a need of over 4000 million units, the availability is 3000 million units. This has led to periodic power cuts and limitation in supply.

Roads and transport are a source of major dissatisfaction. In order to meet the transport needs of the population, the city depends totally on a road-based system. The city has inherited a narrow road system and as a result the older parts of the city have problems in easy movement of vehicles. The land used for the road network is about 17% as compared to 30–33% in cities of the developed countries. Another major constraint is the poor public transport system, which has led to an attendant rise in ownership of private vehicles, from 24/1000 in 1971 to 200/1000 in 1997, mainly due to the increased number of two-wheelers (546% increase), with attendant problems of road congestion. There are two major proposals to overcome the problem—namely the circular rail and overhead rail system. The city is also building its first flyovers this year. The annual public expenditure on health is $3/person/year.

Housing

The average size of the household is 5.7 and this has remained the same over the last three decades. The distribution of households by number of rooms occupied is given in Table 5.3.

During the last decade, there has been an increase in multi-storeyed apartments all over the city, along with an increase in slums. There are about 400 slums in the city, accounting for 12% (over 0.5 million) of the population of the city. The number of slums was not significant in 1970

TABLE 5.3
Distribution of Households by Number of Rooms Occupied

Year	*1 room*	*2 rooms*	*3 rooms*	*4 rooms*	*5 and above*
1971	45.4	27.5	11.9	7.4	7.8
1981	45.0	27.0	12.5	15.5	

(150 slums with around 0.1 million) but currently they are straining on the amenities and act as a barrier in the planned and healthy growth of the city.

Major activities

Bangalore city is considered ideal for setting up industries, due to a favourable industrial climate, available economic infrastructure and the weather. Indian Telephone Industries was the first major public sector industry established in 1948. Apart from public sector units, there are many large scale industries, and about 300 medium to large scale industries in Bangalore, forming 44% of the state total. The number of small scale industries increased from 1100 in 1969–70 to 20,000 in 1990–91.

HISTORY OF MENTAL HEALTH SERVICES

The organisation of mental health services in the city of Bangalore during the last 150 years falls into four phases.

The first phase refers to the period of 1837 to 1937, when a small mental asylum was functioning in the heart of the city. Not much information is available about this phase. The second phase begins with the building of the modern mental hospital in 1937 outside the city. This was built as an open hospital with a pavilion design. This centre was also a pioneer in introducing ECT and psychosurgery around the same time as the rest of the world. The third phase can be traced to the period from 1954 when the All India Institute of Mental Health (AIIMH) was built as the first mental health training centre for the needs of independent India. The AIIMH and the mental hospital worked in cooperation, with the hospital under state control and the Institute under federal support. The beginning of the training courses in psychiatry, clinical psychology and psychiatric nursing in 1954 brought a lot of changes in the hospital. Some of the significant ones were the setting up of daily out-patient services, the specialised services for family therapy, children, persons with drug dependence, rehabilitation, open wards, and neurological services.

In 1974, the hospital and the training institute were combined under one management to form the National Institute of Mental Health and Neuro-Sciences (NIMHANS). In the last 23 years, the Institute has come to be an innovator of a number of mental health initiatives. The Institute is the chief mental health facility in the city.

The fourth phase of mental health activities are of recent origin. These are in the areas of alternative community mental health facilities, initiatives by the voluntary organisations, and both private and public general hospital psychiatric units.

Currently all the major general hospitals in the city have psychiatric units with out-patient departments and in-patient services. The number of private sector psychiatrists is now over 100, compared to a handful less than 40 years back. During the last two decades, the other mental health initiatives have been: (i) school and college mental health programmes, (ii) prison psychiatric services, (iii) suicide prevention, (iv) centres for addiction services, (v) training for staff of institutionalised children and homeless persons. All of these developments have made Bangalore the 'mental health capital' of India. The city has started a large number of innovative activities, to be adopted by other centres in the country.

MENTAL HEALTH SERVICES

All of the services available in the city are accessed by the general population in an 'open' manner. There is no committed system of primary, secondary and tertiary care referral pathways. Similarly, the private and public facilities are used interchangeably. A large factor determining the use of a service is the economic status of the patient. In addition, the reputation of a clinician or hospital also attracts specific groups of patients. There is as yet no attempt to link all the services in the city by any system. It can be observed that there is considerable shopping around and duplication of services by patients. The lack of linkage is a reflection of the lack of a National Health Service-like structure for the urban population.

Facilities

The mental health facilities of the city of Bangalore consist of NIMHANS, medical colleges, private psychiatric facilities, half-way and long-stay homes, drug dependence and learning disability units. The total number of psychiatrists in both public and private sectors is 110 (2.29/100K at risk). The number of clinical psychologists is about 30 and social workers 25. The total number of psychiatric beds is about 900, of which about 400 are being used for Bangalore residents at any one time (8.33/ 100K at risk).

NIMHANS

In addition to providing quality care to patients in both in-patient and out-patient settings, the department of psychiatry has continued its effort of offering specialised services in various areas:

Child and adolescent mental health. The Child and Adolescent Mental Health services provide high standards of care. Its staff members also function as resource persons for various governmental and non-governmental organisations. One such important activity initiated during the year was with the collaboration of a voluntary organisation, SAMVAD. It involved the designing and implementation of an interactive workshop cum survey methodology for researching childhood sexual abuse among girls. This work has subsequently been extended to focus on research issues concerning disclosure, and to formulate strategies for interventions.

Community mental health. The community mental health service has regular activities to provide services to the rural population around Sakalawara, as well as through the neuro-psychiatric extension clinics in five Taluk headquarters. A system of recording and reviewing of the data has been developed. A major new initiative that has been made in collaboration with the faculty of departments—namely clinical psychology, psychiatric social work, and nursing—is the addition of areas (other than severe mental disorders) for future development of programmes. Specifically, the focus has been on understanding and developing interventions at the level of: (i) families of the mentally ill; (ii) developing a mental health programme for the child care workers; (iii) school mental health programme to cover children from primary school to the high school. In each of these areas, the efforts are towards prevention of mental disorders and promotion of mental health in addition to treatment of mentally ill individuals. The staff also provide support to the district mental health programmes in the state of Karnataka.

ECT services. The department has a highly sophisticated clinical service for ECT. Recently, a brief pulse constant current ECT device was added to further augment its services. The physical structure of the ECT service is in accordance with contemporary guidelines.

Addiction treatment services. More than 800 patients receive treatment each year for substance-abuse related problems. In-patient services are available for 60 patients. In-patient care includes a group therapy programme, which is conducted thrice weekly. In addition, family groups are also held weekly. The extension services have been organised with a view to extend consultancy support for more non-governmental organisations.

HIV/AIDS services. This new activity was started in November 1994. The HIV/AIDS clinic runs on Friday afternoons in the Family Psychiatry Centre. Patients attending the clinic are assessed for psychiatric and medical problems and appropriate interventions are offered. The activities of this facility include: (i) pre- and post-test counselling; (ii) crisis intervention for seropositives and their families; (iii) medical assessment and liaison with appropriate agencies; (iv) networking with other governmental and non-governmental agencies for rehabilitation and long-term care; (v) counselling in risk reduction for individuals engaging in high risk behaviours; and (vi) providing information and education to the worried well.

Medical colleges

There are five medical colleges in the city. All of them have separate departments of psychiatry with in-patient and out-patient services. A major activity of the colleges is the training of undergraduates, in addition to providing services.

Private psychiatric facilities

The institutional facility in the private sector consists of one fully specialised psychiatric hospital and a number of general hospital psychiatric units. The amount of in-patient care provided by these units is variable, as most of them use the general beds for the admission of patients.

Addiction treatment facilities

Drug abuse and dependence in the city is almost all related to alcohol dependence. In 1997, a survey of 1680 patients admitted to 11 addiction treatment facilities showed that 97% of the patients were being treated for alcohol dependent problems. Currently, a network of organisations working in this area has been established in the city. A quarterly newsletter links the activities of the centres. The major care programme is detoxification and follow-up care. Specialised rehabilitative services are available in only two centres.

Half-way homes

The growth of these facilities is special to Bangalore city. Nearly 75% of the half-way homes in the country are located in Bangalore. This could be a reflection of the need of people coming to NIMHANS as well as the available support of NIMHANS and other mental health institutions. All of the centres, except for one, are for short duration stay (up to nine months to one year). The focus of work is on social skills training, family therapy, and vocational rehabilitation.

The dates of the establishment of the different half-way homes in the city are listed below:

1.	Medicopastoral Association	1972
2.	Atma Shakti Vidyalaya	1980

3. Richmond Fellowship 1986
4. Puskara After care Home 1987
5. Cadabam's home for the mentally disabled 1994
6. Family fellowship society for psychosocial rehabilitation services 1995
7. Raju Rehabilitation Foundation 1997

Psychological services

The psychological services in the city are only developed to a limited extent. They are now seen as independent professions providing services, along with psychiatrists, or on their own. The common problems for which they provide services are childhood problems, marital problems, adjustment problems and stress-related disorders. They use a wide variety of interventions, including behaviour therapy, psychotherapy, family therapy and group work. The other groups work in some of the selected schools as school counsellors. The majority of the schools and colleges do not have psychological services. Some psychologists work as part of the addiction treatment services. Due to the paucity of personnel, there is a limited number of trained professionals to work in a variety of voluntary initiatives such as those with street children, women's groups, slum dwellers, etc.

Private sector psychiatrists

During the last three decades private sector psychiatry has grown in a big way. The majority of psychiatrists work as individuals and use a wide variety of treatment modalities. A number of professionals working in the government hospitals also work in the evenings in the private sector. An interesting aspect is that the psychiatric specialisation of the private sector psychiatrists is still very limited.

Emergency services

Emergency services are available in all the major hospitals, along with ambulance services. However, there is as yet no 24-hour phone line for psychiatric patients. Emergency care is provided without involving the police in most situations. Of the centres, NIMHANS offers a continuous emergency service.

Community services for the mentally ill

At present there is no committed community level service for the mentally ill. The city of Bangalore was one of the pioneers in initiating the home visiting services of nurses as early as 1978 (Pai & Kapur, 1982). However, this service was only for a limited period and did not extend to all the mentally ill.From centres like NIMHANS, where a significant number of psychiatric social workers are on the staff, they reach out to patients on a case-by-case basis. More recently, an attempt at organising home visiting nurses is being planned by AMEND. As a result the current services are to be accessed by the mentally ill and their families. This leads to variable rates of utilisation of services, more often based on their perception and paying capacity, rather than the real need. The city has been home to some innovative programmes of community services for the terminally ill, elderly persons in small pockets of the population. The needs in these areas are high, but the infrastructure, staff, administrative support and funding are lacking.

Training programmes

The city is host to the biggest postgraduate training centre in the country, namely NIMHANS. There are training programmes for postgraduates in psychiatry, clinical psychology, psychiatric social work and psychiatric nursing. Training programmes for psychiatrists are also available at three other centres, although the numbers trained at these centres every year is small.

In addition, a variety of training programmes for non-specialists are conducted by different institutions. These vary in duration and focus, but cover the whole range of mental health. Some of the important training programs involve training for urban general practitioners, rural medical officers, primary care health workers, parents of mentally retarded persons, clinical psychologists, social workers, school and college teachers, child care workers, staff working with street children, addiction treatment services, prison staff, and staff working with homeless persons.

SPECIALISED FEATURES OF THE SERVICES

From the description of the population of the city and the available services, it is clear that there is a big mismatch between the needs and the services. This disparity has resulted in the development of innovative programmes in the city. The essence of these are: (1) recognition of the needs of the population for mental health services; (2) utilisation of community resources; (3) organisation of services in the non-institutional and community-friendly settings; (4) strengthening of family support; (5) treatment in non-restrictive settings; (6) integration of services, (7) encouragement of community involvement and self-help in the community.

These principles have been reflected in the National Mental Health

Programme (NMHP) for India, formulated in 1982 (Director General of Health Services, 1982). The NMHP has the following objectives:

1. To ensure availability and accessibility of minimum mental health care for all in the foreseeable future, particularly to the most vulnerable and under-privileged sections of the population.
2. To encourage application of mental health knowledge in general health care and in social development.
3. To promote community participation in the mental health service development and to stimulate efforts towards self-help in the community.

The approaches utilised to achieve the goals are:

1. Diffusion of mental health skills to the periphery of the health service system.
2. Appropriate appointment of tasks in mental health care.
3. Equitable and balanced territorial distribution of resources.
4. Integration of basic mental health care into general health services.
5. Linkage to community development.
6. Rehabilitation.
7. Prevention.
8. Mental retardation and drug dependence care.

Of the many special features of the services in the city, three are described here as they (a) reflect a way of enhancing trained manpower, (b) provide least restrictive facilities for the long-term mentally ill and, (c) illustrate how families can join to support each other as well as pressurise administrators to provide the needed services (Nagarajaiah, Chandrasekhar, Murthy, Isaac, & Verma, 1987; Murthy & Wig, 1993).

Integration of mental health with primary care

The basic premise for this approach is the recognition that a major part of the mental health tasks can be better done by primary care personnel. In addition, this is also the reflection of the need to provide services in a friendly, affordable and accessible manner with the least amount of stigma. The approaches have been modified to meet the needs of the rural and urban populations.

Rural services

The rural population of the Bangalore development area has a large population spread out in small villages. On average the size of the population of a village is less than 1000. They have limited access to easy transport and other communications. A striking feature of the needs of the mentally ill is that the majority of them are living with their families but do not receive regular modern treatments. Rehabilitation is based on traditional rural agrarian activities. There is high tolerance of the ill by the community and near total support by the family members.

An innovative approach has been tried in the Solur Area: During the period of 1985–1996 a systematic attempt was made to study the feasibility of integrating mental health with primary health care. As part of this project all the 7 medical officers, 7 health supervisors and 35 junior health assistants were provided skills in recognition, referral, first aid, follow-up and treatment (for doctors) covering a population of 96,600. The mental health care undertaken by them was systematically studied for 18 months both for the amount of care provided and the quality of care. The findings demonstrated the feasibility of mental health care by the primary health care personnel. An important outcome was the finding that for the primary health personnel to continue to provide mental health care they require support and supervision by the mental health professionals at least once a month. This study also resulted in manuals for the different categories of health personnel, training evaluation forms and health education materials. This study also formed the basis for the next phase of a large scale community mental health project for a population unit of 2 million people (Nagarajaiah et al., 1987).

Urban initiatives

In the urban area, people have access not only to the big hospitals but also to the private sector general practitioners (GPs). Since in the city of Bangalore, as in other parts of the country, there is no national health service, a significant proportion utilise the services of the general practitioners in the private sector. It is estimated that about two-thirds of the care is provided by this sector. The initiatives taken in this area have aimed to provide training in essential mental health care for general practitioners. Training for general practitioners has been made available in a range of intensity, and to suit the available time of a wide range of practitioners. The findings of these experiences have been:

1. It has been noted that GPs are generally poor corresponders, responding poorly to postal and/or newspaper communication with a response rate of about 20%. However, they respond more positively on personal contact. This was especially effective when a liaison service was available.
2. A GP tends jealously to protect his unique professional freedom and

dreads to function as an extension or extra pair of hands of specialists.
3. The GP expects their patients to be referred back to their care when they refer patients a specialist's plan of management is often not practicable in the primary care setting of general practice.
4. Neurosis, depression, alcohol-related problems, sexual problems, psychosomatic and somatopsychic problems are overwhelmingly represented in clients of general practice.
5. The GPs seek to acquire practical skills rather than acquire theoretical knowledge.

Training of personnel

A major contribution of Bangalore is the development of training packages for primary health care personnel. These have included manuals, evaluation material, comparison of different types of evaluation and preparation of audio-visual materials. They have demonstrated the feasibility of training doctors in two weeks and health workers in one week. Uniformly the knowledge, attitude and mental health skills were low prior to the training. The training programmes resulted in significant changes in these areas (Sriram, Sundar, Uday, Chandrasekhar, Isaac, & Murthy, 1990; Murthy, 1992).

Manuals

The basic manuals for training of primary care personnel have undergone a lot of changes. Current manuals reflect the needs of the PHC personnel as well as those aspects of care that can be undertaken by them.

The continuous care clinic

This is a weekly clinic set up at NIMHANS to deal with the multiple needs of patients with psychoses of long duration. The same team of professionals provide care. The special efforts are to; (1) maintain a personalised service; (2) limit the waiting period; (3) optimise the pharmacological interventions; (4) educate the patient and families; (5) organise services for needs in the areas of job, marital life and community living. This experience has been found to increase regularity, subjective satisfaction of patients and their families and clinical improvement. It is planned to combine this with home visiting services for the families living in the city. In conclusion, the NIMHANS efforts at integration of mental health with primary health care haves firmly laid the foundation for use of this method as an important approach to meet mental health needs in a situation of limited resources.

The role of voluntary organisations

The Richmond Fellowship Society (India), Bangalore

The Richmond Fellowship Society (India) was established as a Registered Charitable organisation in the year 1986 in Bangalore, at the initiative of the Richmond Fellowship International (RFI). The objects of the Fellowship are:

1. To offer skilled help to those who are chronically mentally and emotionally disturbed and need support to be rehabilitated and re-integrated with the family and community.
2. To create public awareness and to enhance people's understanding of themselves and the disabled.
3. To promote mental health in the community, particularly by providing courses in personality development and humanism, and giving an opportunity to the community to interact with the disabled.
4. To collaborate with all activities of similar organisations.

The first house of the Fellowship 'Vikas' (which means 'to blossom'), was a trial project and was set up in farm land made available by the family members of M.M. Farms. This house was to provide residential care facilities for 10 male residents. To support this endeavour, the RF International provided a coordinator, who was a professional, to run this facility. Encouraged by the success of Vikas, two years later the RF headquarters secured financial assistance to set up a model house to accommodate 21 residents. This house was called 'ASHA' (meaning 'hope') and is deliberately placed in a residential area, the aim being to provide as close a proximity as possible to the larger community. The style in these two houses is basically informal, although day-to-day life is organised by a structured programme. This reflects the ordinary pattern of an average household. However, rehabilitative activities form the core programme. Regular habits are inculcated by setting times of getting up, personal care, meals and other activities, because many residents have been incapacitated so far as normal routines are concerned. The whole morning for five days each week is geared to a work activity programme. Occupational therapy activities are set to individual needs and help residents develop a number of skills and the habit of work itself. The emphasis is on group life. Residents also have individual counselling sessions with their keyworker on the staff team. Families are involved from the very inception of placing their wards in the process, in family therapy, and in a 3-monthly progress review.

Referrals to these houses are made by psychiatrists. The family and the applicant are invited to stay for a trial period ranging from 3–7 days. This gives him or her a chance to experience what the house is like, and then to make a decision to live in the community. Since the establishment of the Fellowship, over 300 residents have received rehabilitation programmes, and are drawn from all over the country and from neighbouring countries.

Staff. Staffing being the crucial ingredient by which the therapeutic community stands or falls, a staff member of the therapeutic community house has to be a 'jack of all trades'. Staff members have to be therapeutic, not only in their personalities and professional discipline, but also in their daily living. Hence the RFI training is formulated to train and support the staff to stay on this job. Each house has a staff team of one staff member for at least 3–4 residents. Their role is to encourage positive interaction between community members, to give support to individual residents and to carry the final responsibility in the welfare of the whole household. They keep in touch with the residents, family, and the psychiatrist, as and when necessary. The staff are also responsible for the day-to-day administration of the home. They come with the background qualification of clinical psychology, or of medical psychiatric social work, and also receive training under the training programme of the Fellowship. They are also supported by volunteers coming from the local area and volunteers are a link with the local community.

Training programme. There is no other training centre in India with the emphasis on the therapeutic community approach. The Richmond Fellowship International placed a training office for a period of two years to start a training programme in Bangalore. In 1989 an in-service training programme was organised by the RFI with its staff who are already working in the two houses. This was a 10-month course with 2-hour sessions twice a week. Based on this experience, the RFI (India) modified the duration of the course of the in-service programme from 10 months to 4 months. The training programme is now held once a year and is of 6 months duration. From 1989 to 1995 the Fellowship has trained 39 para-professionals. The trainees come from different parts of India.

Medical Pastoral Association (MPA)

The Medical Pastoral Association (MPA) in Bangalore was founded in 1964 by a small group of dedicated men and women, members of St Mark's Cathedral, pastors, doctors and other caring professionals, and lay persons. MPA was one of the first voluntary organisations in the country concerned about the physical, mental and spiritual dimensions of the health of individuals, their families and the whole community. MPA, an autonomous non-profit secular body, was registered in 1972 under the Mysore Societies Registration Act of 1960.

The initial work of MPA was with alcoholics and with people who had attempted suicide. MPA has trained several batches of concerned people in suicide awareness and how to help depressed people. The Managing Committee of MPA strongly felt the need to help in the rehabilitation of partially recovered mentally ill persons, as no such facility existed at that time. In 1978, the Half-Way Home for recovering mentally persons was opened—the first in India, placed in the general community.

The Half-Way Home. The Half-Way Home is a big cottage comprising six rooms with three beds in each, another room for the female staff to reside in, one for the house parents' office, three halls (for occupational therapy, recreation and dining), a kitchen and a store. The Administrative Block is double-storied and includes the Bangalore Mental Health Information Centre. The Half-Way Home (HWH) is a transitional home and not a psychiatric treatment facility. It has the atmosphere of a big home with house-parents, staff and fellow residents who mingle easily and know each other well. Patients who have been treated in psychiatric hospitals or by psychiatrists are carefully screened by MPA's consulting psychiatrists at NIMHANS and then interviewed by the Admissions Committee consisting of a secretary, administrator, house-parents, and senior counsellor. They are admitted on the condition that their medication is stabilised, and they are ready for the HWH programmes. The duration of stay is 9 to 12 months.

Staffing. An administrator is in charge of administrative aspects, including the routine office work, with the help of an accountant, typist and an attender. A mature and experienced couple are employed by MPA to be the house-parents to see to the day-to-day running of the MPA, and are in charge of the helping staff—cooks, gardener, etc. The counselling staff are recruited from MA degree holders in clinical psychology or social work. They are employed by MPA, generally full-time, and occasionally part-time. There are usually about 4 counsellors for about 20 residents. Some of the counsellors reside on the campus and take turns to do the duties of the house-parents on their day off. A warden is appointed to look after the hostel. Staff members get regular in-service training, attend conferences and share experience with others in the field. There are also special team building sessions to help avoid burn-out.

Community support. There is a remarkable contribution from the community in Bangalore who participate in the organisational activities. At the Annual General Body Meeting of MPA, the members of the Management

Committee are elected—dedicated volunteers from all walks of life. In addition to helping office bearers in making major decisions, most members are chairpersons of standing committees and participate in programmes. There is strong support from doctors of NIMHANS, who make both organisational and individual personal contributions in running the HWH and helping to organise public programmes.

Methodology. Activities at the HWH are designed to improve specific deficit areas of the residents. A structured time-table is drawn up and residents are required to follow it and attend all programmes. Common problems seen in most residents when they are first admitted are a lack of volition, inability to get up in the morning, little or no personal hygiene, no interest in activities, reluctance to take medication. They are generally slow and lethargic. Problems of irritability and aggressiveness may erupt unexpectedly, and staff members have to learn to deal with each crisis using their own expertise. Self-pity, depression, suspiciousness, boredom, inability to make confident decisions are also problems to be tackled. This is done in a loving, caring, yet disciplined manner by the entire HWH community and through a systematic range of therapies—occupational, art, play, music, group therapies, and individual counselling. Independent living skills and social skills have to be learned. Programmes at HWH for mental stimulation include 'Quiz' and 'Current Affairs'—reading of newspapers is encouraged so that they are aware of the outside world. Classes in English and value education are conducted. For physical stimulation, aerobics, games, gardening, and walking are encouraged. Yoga helps to calm their inner agitation. Art in various forms and using clay in pottery is found to have healing properties. Cooking is also a rewarding programme.

Besides this, regular outings are organised for the residents—movies, restaurants, exhibitions, to teach them responsibility, handling money and mixing in the community. The residents are expected to be rehabilitated sufficiently within one year to return to their families or to take up jobs to support themselves and live independently. The current occupancy of the HWH is 25 residents. MPA also provides a day-care facility where a person can attend all the programmes and return home each evening.

The hostel. The Navjeevan Hostel, a two-storied building with eight rooms with three beds in each was opened in 1988 on the same campus as the HWH. This Hostel is for residents who, after completing their rehabilitation programme of about one year at HWH, are functional enough to hold a job (full-time or part-time) or are undergoing vocational training in an external location. After a stressful day at work, returning to a safe and caring environment where counsellors are available by appointment, instils a sense of security and independence in the hostel-dwellers. There were practical problems in working women residents staying in the same hostel, especially as supervision is minimal. The self-help initiative promotes a friendly and familiar environment for the suffering families to gain from the experience of others.

The contribution of users and carers

AMEND

This is a self-help group for users and carers, started in borrowed premises with borrowed furniture. In the words of the founder (Mrs Nirmala Srinivasan):

> Since 1992, the membership has been growing slowly but steadily. Today, it has a strength of around 70 families. 'When we met for the first meeting, even though we had not met each other, we felt we knew each other'. Our experiences were sufficient to lay the foundations. The emotional bonding is our first and foremost commitment. In fact, some families are not able to appreciate because they are in the trap of misconceptions and myths about schizophrenia. For these families, emotional support or sharing and learning comes last in the agenda. The day-to-day agony of going through with patient drives them unwillingly to look for long-term institutionalisation. The families of the mentally ill need help. Some of the storms that can sweep over the families when schizophrenia strikes are: sorrow, fear, disruption of family relationships, disruption of family health, despair, anxiety, guilt, difficulty in accepting the illness, a feeling of isolation, exhaustion of spirit and resources, and apprehension about the future. There are hundreds of families who need help. Someone they love is suffering from schizophrenia. But these families are isolated. They need to meet and find emotional companionship. New demands were made on the members to guide each other and share each other's experiences with a view to learn about various aspects of coping with the stress—a problem about which they know almost nothing. Mental health educational programmes are aimed at normal people coping with normal stress problems. The affected families become aware of the facts the hard way after living with the ill person for a number of years. The self-help initiatives promote a friendly and familiar environment for the suffering families to gain from the experience of others.

From one stage to another, AMEND gained strength. Emotional support and shared learning led to participants feeling for each other. The AMEND family is always there to help in a crisis. It became a way of hope to all of us. In almost all the meetings, the repeated emphasis is on what the families can do to promote the well-being of the patient, and prevent crisis and further deterioration. Many families have had exposure from those who have benefited from family therapy services. It was also found that the attendance of the meetings varies with the agenda. Lectures from leading psychiatrists attracted the maximum crowd; similarly, any input on long-term care and rehabilitation was also well attended. The crux of this successful transaction between families lay in the fact that they all shared the same agony which the professionals can only talk about.

Besides self-support, information dissemination was the next major landmark in AMEND's modest achievements. With the immense support given by professional psychiatrists, psychiatric social workers and other NGOs, AMEND reached a stage where the focus had shifted from illness *per se*, to its management. New members who come with the hope of finding instant solutions, are encouraged to look into the benefits of multi-therapy treatment models, and not get bogged down with the conventional syndrome of chronicity of schizophrenia. Knowledge of the new drugs, such as clozapine, have raised hopes, pushing the agenda into action plans. Similarly, AMEND is also trying to get the term 'Disability' redefined so as to make the benefits of the disabled available to the mentally ill, under the Persons with Disability Act of India (1995).

Based on the experience of AMEND, it can be said that self-help groups can go a long way in educating the public, raising funds for research, and fighting for better legislation. They can lend emotional support to families. Families no longer need feel isolated. Talking to others helps. Relatives see their secrecy and come forward to admit they have a problem. Many times a mentally ill person creates havoc in family relationships. Compassionate counselling by trained therapists arranged by self-help groups can lead to meaningful relationships again. Friction between husband and wife as to how to handle a crisis is turned into a supportive effort by the parents to deal with the matter in an emotionally restrained way.

THE FUTURE

The city of Bangalore has more psychiatric treatment facilities than other cities of India. In addition, there are a wide variety of community facilities; such as day care centres, half way homes, drug dependence facilities and suicide prevention centres. There are also a number of mental health promotion activities like school mental health programmes, stress management courses and mental health education activities. In addition, NIMHANS Bangalore; has been a source of training of manpower, provider of new mental health information and support to the wide variety of community initiatives. However, today, there are a number of areas where there are lacunae: (1) the services are not geographically spread out for easy accessibility; (2) the numbers are far less than the total need; (3) the many initiatives, like self-help groups, are of recent origin; (4) there is no community support at home level by visiting nurses or other professionals for the majority of the mentally ill, or elderly persons; (5) there are as yet no new community centres for socio-cultural activities other than those related to religious places of worship; (6) no significant attempts have been made to involve religious leaders in promotion of mental health; (7) parental skills programmes are yet to begin in the city on a regular basis; (8) monitoring of the mental health aspects of the city is yet to occur; (9) the influencing of policies of the city by the mental health professionals is not significant; (10) the planners have not recognised mental health as an important aspect of the city plans. All these are areas for future initiatives.

The population of Bangalore is expected to grow to between 5.7 million and 6.2 million by the year 2001 (Bhattacharjee & Yadav, 1993). Urban life has many advantages and disadvantages for those living in the city. For the mentally ill individuals and their families, the disadvantages are even more challenging. Though the families and ill members have wider availability of services, they are not always accessible or affordable. In contrast, they lose out on the support of a homogeneous, large kinship network of rural life, as well as the simple life of the rural areas (Shankar, 1994). It is clear that many new services will be required to deal with the needs of a larger city, and much of the burden is likely to fall upon voluntary organisations like the Richmond Fellowship. The Fellowship has plans to extend the facilities to other areas as well. These include:

1. Setting up of half-way homes in other parts of the country in association with voluntary organisations, the guidelines for which have been laid down by the Governing Council of the Fellowship.
2. Group Home: From 2nd October 1995, the Fellowship started a Group Home facility (long stay home) 'Jyothi' ('Light') at the request of several families. The guidelines wereprovided by the professionals discussed at the Symposium on 'Long Term Care for Chronic Schizophrenic Patients' held in May 1994. This facility is established very close to Asha and can accommodate 12 residents.
3. Day Care Centre with a vocational training facility. The Fellowship has received nearly 1900 m^2 of land on a 99 year lease basis from a philanthropist. The Government of Karnataka has permitted to set up the centre on this land. This centre will also house a training college and library and it is proposed to set up one more half-way home in the land available there. The total estimated cost of this project is about Rs.62 lakhs (£100,000) for the building alone.
4. A low cost rural project for rehabilitation of the mentally ill, 60 km from Bangalore is being processed. The emphasis will be on rural based technology of sericulture, horticulture, floriculture, including utilising the facilities at the Industrial Training Institute. It is also

proposed to enlist the support of the families of this village for providing expenses for this half-way home on a sharing basis—i.e. one day expenses by each family.

For the mental health professionals, the challenges of creating a mentally healthy city are many, and cover provision of services, prevention of mental disorders and promotion of mental health (Wig & Murthy, 1994). Further integration of mental health services with primary care will be necessary, together with the provision of mental health facilities in the community such as day care centres, half-way homes and rehabilitation facilities. There will need to be an expansion of services in the community to provide support for families and persons with mental illnesses. The changing age structure of the population will require increased support and networking for the elderly. School mental health services might be expanded, with the provision of parental skills training. User's organisations might provide self-help groups of 'at risk' individuals. There need; to be decentralised services for marginalised people, for example, street children and slum dwellers. Religious leaders should be involved in the promotion of mental health. At a public health level there needs to be more mental health education to decrease the stigma attached to mental disorders, as well as monitoring the mental health of the city population. These are great challenges, but the past leadership taken by the Bangalore city in mental health would be expected to take up the challenges of the future.

REFERENCES

Bhattacharjee, P.J. & Yadav S.S. (1993). *Consequences of a fast growing metropolis: a case study of Bangalore centre.* (Mimoo pages 155). Bangalore: Population Centre.

Director General of Health Services (1982). *National Mental Health Programme for India.* New Delhi: Ministry of Health and Family Welfare.

Gazettes of India (1990). *Bangalore District.* Karnataka State.

Murthy, S.R. (1992). Mental health. In A. Mukhopadhyah (Ed.), *State of India's Health* (pp. 400–414). New Delhi: Voluntary Health Association of India.

Murthy, R. & Wig, N.N. (1993). Evaluation of the progress in mental health in India since independence. In P.P. Mane & K.Y. Gandevia (Eds), *Mental Health in India—Issues and Concerns* (pp. 387–405). Bombay: Tata Institute of Social Sciences.

Nagarajaiah, Chandrasekhar C.R., Murthy, S.R., Isaac, M.K., Parthasarathy, R., Verma, M. (1987). Relevance and methods of training multipurpose health workers in delivery of basic mental health care. *Indian Journal of Psychiatry, 29*, 161–164.

Pai, S. & Kapur, R.L. (1982). Impact on treatment intervention on the relationship between the dimensions of clinical psychopathology, social dysfunction and burden on families of schizophrenic patients. *Psychological Medicine. 12*, 651–658.

Population Crisis Committee (1990). *Cities: Life in the world's 100 largest metropolitan areas.* Washington: Population Reference Bureau.

Shankar, R. (1994). Interventions with families of people with schizophrenia in India. In A.B.

Hatfield (Ed.), *Family Interventions in Mental Illness* (*New Directions for Mental Health Services No. 62*) (pp. 79–88). San Francisco: Jossey-Bas.

Sriram, T.G., Sundar, M., Uday, K.G.S., Chandrasekhar, C.R., Isaac, M.K., Murthy, S. R. (1990). Training of primary health care medical officers in mental health care—Errors in clinical judgment before and after training. *General Hospital Psychiatry, 12*, 384–389.

Wig, N.N. & Murthy, S.R. (1994). From mental illness to mental health. *Health for the Millions, 20*, 2–4.

CHAPTER SIX

Mental health in the city of Copenhagen, Denmark

Marianne C. Kastrup
Copenhagen University Hospital, Hvidovre, Denmark

THE CITY OF COPENHAGEN

General characteristics

Copenhagen is the capital of Denmark. Within the boundaries of the municipality of Copenhagen an independent municipality, Frederiksberg, is located with approximately 90,000 inhabitants.

Social characteristics

The city has a number of industries such as breweries, electronic and pharmaceutical industries. The city houses the largest university in Denmark, the University of Copenhagen, which is a state university. Moreover, the city houses a number of other educational institutions, such as The Royal Veterinarian and Agricultural University, The Technical University, The Music Academy, The Academy of Fine Arts, and The School of Economics and Business Administration. The city has a sea port and an airport. The airport is the main airport for all the Scandinavian countries, and both ports are related to the fact that Copenhagen has a rather large tourist industry.

Social problems. The city of Copenhagen is faced with a range of social problems. The population is skewed with an overrepresentation of elderly and single persons. In the inner city there is a small population of homeless people some of whom live as bag ladies, others live in various types of hostels. A large proportion of this population suffers from mental disorders. The city has a concentration of persons exhibiting problems with alcohol as well as other substance abuses.

Copenhagen also comprises a large immigrant population concentrated in certain areas of the city. This concentration has consequences both for the school populations—resulting in high proportions of immigrant/non-Danish speaking children—and for gang crimes.

Population statistics

Copenhagen had its peak population of 668,105 inhabitants in 1950, but subsequently the population has slowly decreased to the present population of 471,300. The average expected lifetime, in the region of Copenhagen, in the period 1988–89 amounted to 68.2 years in men and 75.6 years in women. The average life expectancy is lower in Copenhagen than in the counties surrounding the city.

The total foreign population in the city amounted in 1995 to 44,661; of which the largest group, namely 15,550, originated from Africa and Asia, 12,130 had origins in Europe outside the EC and Scandinavia, 7911 originated from EC countries, and 5169 originated from other Scandinavian countries. The remaining originated from other areas of the world.

The unemployment rate for the population with residence in the municipality of Copenhagen is 14.2% of the registered labour force, compared to an unemployment rate of 10% of the entire Copenhagen region including neighbouring counties. A total of 18.7% of the male population in the municipality has experienced unemployment, compared to an average of 12.1% in the Copenhagen area. In women the corresponding figures amounted to 15.1% in the municipality of Copenhagen and 11.9% in the Copenhagen region.

The enrollment capacity of institutions for children and young people showed in the municipality of Copenhagen that 48.7 per 100 inhabitants were enrolled, compared to 40.4 in the Copenhagen region as a whole. The city had a lower proportion of children in municipal preschool classes with 73% of 6-year-olds in Copenhagen compared to 85% in the Copenhagen region as a whole.

The population of the municipality of Copenhagen showed relatively less affinity with the state church than the Copenhagen region as a whole. Among children born in 1992 51.7% were baptised compared to 67.5% in the entire region. Of those that married 47.3% in the municipality of

Copenhagen were married in a church compared to 51.4% in the whole region. The proportion of the population that paid church tax amounted to 77.6% in comparison with 82.5% in the whole region.

Copenhagen is a relatively deprived area measured by the average income and allowance. Thus the average income and allowance for taxable persons were calculated to 119,500 D.kr., compared to 139,600 D.kr. in the region as a whole. Considering the relative distribution of taxable persons, the same tendency appeared as Copenhagen had a relatively larger proportion showing a low income and a relatively small proportion of persons with a high income compared to the region as a whole.

Furthermore, the citizens in the municipality showed relatively less use of their democratic rights in the local-/regional elections as the percentage voting in Copenhagen was relatively small when compared to the neighbouring municipalities. The same was the case for the election to the Danish Parliament, where only 80.1% of the Copenhagen citizens, compared to 84.2% of the region as a whole, voted at the last election (Statistical Yearbook, 1995).

Social services

Denmark has an elaborate social system providing social benefits for citizens in need. The '*Bistandslov*' (Social Help Act) from 1976 is the legislative body regulating the provision of social services that are administered by and under the responsibility of the local municipality.

Copenhagen is divided into 14 boroughs, or social districts, each with its own social district centre, but all under the responsibility of the social magistrate of the municipality. In order to rank the districts according to severity of social problems the following indicators have been used:

1. The number of unemployed age 16–66.
2. The proportion of inhabitants receiving social benefits age 18–44.
3. The proportion of early receivers of pension i.e. prior to the age of 67.
4. The proportion of inhabitants with a total income below 100,000 D.kr. in 1990.

Similarly, the boroughs have been ranked according to their use of psychiatric in-patient care. A comparison of the two rankings showed that the five boroughs ranked as having the greatest social problems were identical with those with the relatively highest use of psychiatric hospital care (Sundhedsdirektoratet, 1993). Each social district centre is responsible for a variety of services, including home help, meals-on-wheels, and district nurses.

To assess health issues in cases presented to the social district centre, each social district receives consultation services from a general practitioner (GP) and a specialist in psychiatry.

GENERAL HEALTH SERVICES

Primary health care

In Denmark, the GP plays a key role in the coordination of the various medical interventions with contact between the patient, relatives, the local network, and other health and social services. All citizens are entitled to a GP and usually they enroll on the list of a GP close to their residence.

The GP also plays a central role in the diagnosis, treatment, and follow-up of psychiatric illness, as a substantial proportion of all contacts having a psychological aspect will not be referred any further, but will be treated in primary care. In relation to hospital care, the GP will in particular be involved when a patient is discharged, as the responsible coordinator of the various therapeutic activities. The GP also refers the patient to secondary institutional care or to private specialists.

The city of Copenhagen has appointed a number of GPs as liaison officers, with the aim of facilitating collaboration between primary and secondary health services, each of whom has responsibility to promote the interaction between a specific department and the GPs in its catchment area.

Other possibilities for help in the community

The social services have various institutions that provide services for the mentally ill people, such as special housing for mentally ill, welfare institutions for socially deprived persons, for homeless persons, and a variety of day centres for the mentally ill. In the city there is ample opportunity to receive psychological help. The limitation is, however, the fact that such consultations usually have to be paid by the patient without possibility for reimbursement. Partial support from the National Health Service for psychological help related to various forms of crisis intervention was established in 1992 on a project basis.

Specialists in psychiatry

A number of specialists in psychiatry provide services independently of psychiatric institutions. These specialists usually work in their own clinic and receive patients referred from GPs. The service provided will typically be free of charge, covered by the National Health Service, but with a limit on the annual number of consultations thus provided. Psychiatrists in private practice in Copenhagen in 1993 numbered 30, of whom 13 were full-time.

Institutional psychiatric care

According to Danish legislation, health services—as opposed to social services—are the responsibility of the regional authorities (counties); with the exception of Copenhagen, which has status as both municipal and regional authority. The municipality of Copenhagen is responsible for the overall health services, and the local politicians have the political and economic responsibility for the quality and level of services. All medical services are free of charge and financed by the taxation system.

DEVELOPMENT OF PSYCHIATRIC SERVICES IN DENMARK

The first hospital for psychiatric patients was established in 1816 in the Sankt Hans Hospital, located approximately 30 km from the city of Copenhagen. At that time the provision of a ward for the mentally ill was considered a task for the local municipality, but no municipality apart from Copenhagen had the funds to carry out this task.

In the light of this, the Danish state took the initiative to establish the necessary institutions for the mentally ill, and at the turn of the century the state took the total responsibility for the psychiatric hospitals and gave the municipality of Copenhagen compensation for running its own mental health service system. Apart from the psychiatric hospital, the city of Copenhagen established psychiatric departments at some of its general hospitals to provide acute and short-term treatment. Patients requiring longer admissions were transferred to the psychiatric hospital.

The development of community mental health services

In 1976, the responsibility for psychiatric services was transferred from the state to the regional authorities (counties). The principle of a sectorised psychiatry emerged concomitantly with the change from state to regional responsibility, and has remained almost unchanged as a main organisational principle.

Over the last decade Denmark has further experienced the development of a variety of community psychiatric services. Several different models have been developed, but each sharing some of the same principles: that community care should focus on multidisciplinary teams with easy accessibility and continuity of care and with a low threshold for referral; that extramural activites, including the establishment of social networks, have a high priority; and that evaluative and preventive aspects should play a central role.

Copenhagen offers extensive community psychiatric care.

Radical changes have thus taken place over the last decade, with an extensive increase in the extramural care, out-patient care as well as community psychiatric care, and with a drastic decrease in the number of psychiatric beds provided.

Mental health services in Copenhagen

Three major plans for the mental health services in the municipality of Copenhagen have been developed in the last decade. The plans from 1987 (Direktoratet for Københavns Hospitalsvaesen, 1987) and 1993 (Sundhedsdirektoratet, 1993) concentrate on the services offered by the municipality of Copenhagen, whereas the last plan from 1996 (Sygehusplan H: S 2000, 1996) was based on the development in 1995 of a new concept, the Copenhagen Hospital Corporation, comprising the services offered by the municipalities of Copenhagen and Frederiksberg.

The psychiatric plan of 1987

In 1987, the city published its psychiatric plan for the years 1988–2000. The city had at that time three psychiatric departments located at three general hospitals: Kommunehospitalet, with 32 beds; Bispebjerg Hospital, with 101 beds; Rigshospitalet, with 55–60 beds.

Further, the mental hospital, Skt. Hans Hospital, had 923 beds used for long-term treatment. The overall objectives of the psychiatric plan for the city were as follows (Direktoratat for Københavns Hospitalsvaesen, 1987):

1. To reorganize the psychiatric mental health care in order to provide more effective support at an earlier point to patients with mental disorders in their own surroundings. It is to be expected that a number of psychiatric disorders may thereby be minimised, if not prevented, and patients enabled to function as far as possible on their own.
2. To organise psychiatry in such a way that treatment will be the least invasive possible for the patients concerned.
3. To promote collaboration between GPs and hospital services in order to support the work of the GPs in the area of psychiatry and to collaborate with the private practising psychiatrists in the organisation of community psychiatry.
4. To extend the existing collaboration between the psychiatric health

services and the activities that take place in private or semi-public regimen aiming to support persons with psychiatric problems, e.g. by strengthening their own social networks.

5. To provide more suitable frames for collaboration regarding the individual patients between the health and social services.
6. To expand the liaison psychiatric services related to general hospitals, thereby improving and facilitating collaboration between psychiatric and general health care.
7. To establish specialised treatment of certain patient categories.
8. To work for the deinstitutionalisation of psychiatry by the transferral of treatment capacity from the psychiatric hospital to smaller units in the city of Copenhagen and by extending extramural care.
9. To improve the physical conditions of the psychiatric services.
10. To strengthen research and developmental activities in the field of psychiatry.
11. To strengthen recruitment and general staff policy within the field of psychiatry, thereby creating better working conditions for health personnel.
12. To establish and improve available offers for further education of psychiatric staff.

Main proposals of the psychiatric plan. In order to reach the above-mentioned goals the psychiatry plan for the city of Copenhagen includes a number of proposals (Sundhedsdirektoratet, 1993) among which the following deserve mention:

1. The present allocation of resources to psychiatry should be maintained in the years to come. Psychiatry should be exempt from any reductions in the health budget that may be brought forward.
2. The psychiatric services should be organised in such a way that acute and general psychiatry should be taken care of by the psychiatric departments placed at general hospitals.
3. The aim should be that at a given general hospital the psychiatric department has the same catchment area as the other hospital departments.
4. The psychiatric departments at the general hospitals should be reorganised in such a way that each unit should serve the same catchment area as a specific community mental health centre, with which the unit should establish close collaboration.
5. Establish community psychiatric centres in the entire municipality of Copenhagen each with a catchment area of between 25,000–55,000 inhabitants. Based upon the evaluation of the first two pilot centres the remaining community psychiatric centres will be organised.

6. The number of beds at the psychiatric hospital should be reduced and the hospital should gradually be reorganised in order to provide care for clearly defined patient categories.
7. Special attention should be given to the future integration of child psychiatry and adolescent psychiatry, with a focus on the coordination between hospital, social and school authorities.
8. The programme for establishing better physical conditions at the psychiatric departments for psychiatric patients should be carried out.
9. As one of the University Hospitals in the city of Copenhagen in 1987 did not have a psychiatric department, such a department should be established.
10. A steering committee should be established in order to provide a fast expansion in the number of collectives and other housing establishments for psychiatric patients.
11. Special courses should be provided for all staff seeking employment at a psychiatric department in order to prepare them for their tasks. Furthermore, post-graduate training of staff working in psychiatry should be continuously provided.
12. A specific post-graduate training for nurses in mental health should be established.

Assumptions for the psychiatry plan. In the psychiatry plan (Sundhedsdirektoratet, 1993) an overall objective was to enlarge treatment capacity through a reorganisation of psychiatric care from in-patient to out-patient care. Consequently, a reduction in the total number of beds does not necessarily reflect a reduction in the treatment capacity within mental health care.

Gerontopsychiatry. The demographic development in the municipality of Copenhagen shows, as mentioned above, a general reduction in the population, with a continuous reduction in the number of elderly people with psychiatric disorders. Furthermore, it is anticipated that elderly patients with light or moderate psychiatric disorders will be increasingly integrated into the normal nursing homes, and not specific psychiatric nursing institutions. The combination of increased out-patient and day hospital care, together with an expansion of community help and nursing, will result in an increasing proportion of elderly people with minor psychiatric disorders remaining in their own homes, instead of being admitted (Sundhedsdirektoratet, 1993).

Community psychiatry in Copenhagen

A main element in the psychiatry plan (Direktoratet for Københavns Hospitalsvaesen, 1987) was the proposal to introduce community psychiatry in the entire municipality of Copenhagen. As early as 1981 it was suggested to introduce community psychiatry, and the proposal to establish two pilot community mental health centres as a first step towards introduction of community psychiatry was discussed in the City Council in 1987.

A main objective in establishing community psychiatry was a wish to allow the patient to remain as much as possible in known surroundings, and to support and treat the patient in the local setting. The idea is also to keep patients out of institutions, to treat them in the vicinity of their home, to help strengthen the local social support systems, and to facilitate the collaboration between the community mental health team, the local social centre and the primary health care system. Ultimately, the hope was to help prevent the emergence or exacerbation of psychiatric problems.

Prior to the introduction of community mental health care it was decided that the community centres should primarily concentrate their work on adult psychiatric patients, and that admissions should not take place in the centres, which would be open in normal working hours. Furthermore, the centres were meant primarily to deal with the more chronic psychiatric population, offering:

1. Assessment of referred patients.
2. Out-patient treatment including psychopharmacological treatment, various psychotherapeutic approaches, supporting and strengthening social networks.
3. Day-centre activity including access to various workshops in order to stimulate patient activities.

The idea was that the staff working at the centres would be multidisciplinary, with each group utilising their specific abilities. The number of community mental health care centres in the city should, when fully established, equal the number of local social districts and each should have a catchment population around 25,000–55,000 (Direktoratet for Københavns Hospitalsvaesen, 1987).

Evaluation of community mental health centres

The services of the first two community mental health centres have been thoroughly evaluated by a group of researchers attached to the University of Copenhagen (Knudsen, Jessen-Petersen, Klitgaard, Krasnik, Nordentoft & Saelan, 1992). The evaluation took place two years after the establishment of the centres. Among the main findings are the following:

1. Establishment of community mental health has only to a very limited degree replaced in-patient treatment.

2. The core group for the community mental health centres have been adults with psychotic disorders, in particular of a chronic nature, and the centres have been able to reach a group of persons with psychotic disorders who have not previously received any treatment.
3. A group of patients with long-term contact with psychiatric services, and who previously were admitted for long periods of time, have been able to manage without admissions thanks to the community mental health centres. The quality of life and satisfaction of this particular group also seem to have improved.
4. As regards the number of staff and the type of staff, services in community psychiatry should be organised in order to utilise available resources at an optimum, and it should be recommended to recruit staff, that have been working at the hospital department related to a given centre.
5. The evaluation showed that within the city of Copenhagen there are differences with regard to demographic distribution, level of psychiatric morbidity, and that the establishment of community mental health centres should take such differences into consideration.
6. Close collaboration between community mental health and general practice and social services should be given high priority.

As regards the balance between community mental health and in-patient care, the introduction of such centres did not automatically lead to a reduction in the need for in-patient care and there seemed no sign of a reduced need of this type of care. Such facts need to be taken into consideration when developing further the psychiatric services, and it is emphasised that a further allocation of resources from in-patient to extramural care may lead to difficulties (Knudsen, Jessen-Petersen, Klitgaard, Krasnik, & Nordentoft et al., 1992).

THE PSYCHIATRIC PLAN OF 1993

The City Council of Copenhagen revised the psychiatry plan of 1987 emphasising two main points (Sundhedsdirektoratet, 1993):

1. Strengthening the collaboration between the health services and the social services by providing maximal social support as early as possible.
2. Re-evaluating the balance between community mental health and stationary psychiatric care.

The overall aim of the revised plan was to provide living conditions for citizens with mental disorders which approached as far as possible those of the normal population. Particular emphasis should be given to patients with various kind of abuse. During the last years, a number of initiatives focusing on the social aspects have materialised, including special housing, temporary and permanent, for citizens with mental problems, day centres, various types of cafés and activity centres. Furthermore, leisure and culture activities have been established.

A new concept in the social services was introduced, namely that of a support & contact person. This person's primary task was to support persons with severe mental disorders in managing their daily life. Such help could include acting as a liaison between the patient and various authorities, landlords, neighbours, GPs, etc. Ideally, this person would make contact with the patient during admission, and plan for the social rehabilitation following discharge. This intensified interaction between health and social services (which also occurs on a more concrete routine level with the aid of a treatment plan) should support patients who have a great need for both social rehabilitation and for the structuring of daily living.

Another new initiative was the development of social 'acting plans' for this vulnerable group of patients, with the aim that close collaboration between health and social services should ensure that the psychiatric treatment plan and the social acting plan are compatible. Based upon the evaluation of the community mental health centres (Knudsen et al., 1992), the psychiatry plan of 1993 also stated that in future community mental health centres should recommend the core group to be persons with severe mental disorders (in particular psychoses of a chronic nature) who are in need of long-term care. Patients with other kinds of mental disorders could be treated only to the extent that the centre has extra capacity. The plan further suggests the establishment of a psychiatric ambulance service, at least on a project basis.

Organisation of psychiatric care

The overall organisation of the mental health services in Copenhagen did not change with the revision of the plan. Thus the hospital-based psychiatric services include:

1. Emergency psychiatric clinic open 24 hours.
2. In-patient facilities for shorter or longer periods.
3. Day hospital services related to psychiatric departments.
4. Out-patient treatment related to the psychiatric departments.
5. Community mental health clinics providing out-patient and day-patient service.

Capacity of the psychiatric departments. In 1993 the municipality of Copenhagen had the following psychiatric departments: Hvidovre Hospital established in 1989; 120 beds), Bispebjerg Hospital (99 beds), Kommune Hospitalet (72 beds), Rigshospitalet (52 beds), and The Psychiatric Hospital (Skt.Hans) (525 beds).

The psychiatric hospital comprised departments for forensic patients, for patients with problems of abuse, for younger psychotics, for long-term care and for general psychiatry. Over the years, the role of this particular hospital has been thoroughly discussed, with the issue of having general psychiatric beds at the psychiatric hospital being particularly debated. It is generally agreed that a specialisation of care, such as forensic psychiatric services or services for patients with abuse, could benefit from special departments at the psychiatric hospital; but on the other hand it may be less evident why the hospital should continue to have departments with general psychiatric care in the light of the fact that the general psychiatric departments cover the entire city.

Treatment plans for individual patients

As part of the Mental Health Act from 1989 the Danish National Board of Health has laid down guidelines regarding treatment plans for patients admitted to psychiatric departments. Within one week of admission a treatment plan should be available, comprising a description of the present symptomatology, the need for further investigations and therapeutic interventions. The treatment plan should comprise information about medical as well as social interventions, together with both short and long-term treatment goals, the approval by the patient and the date for renewal of the treatment plan. For patients with an extended need for various kinds of social interventions, the psychiatry plan of 1993 suggests that the collaboration between health and social services with respect to the social aspect of the treatment plan should be intensified. The idea is to outline this plan during the admission in close collaboration with the user of psychiatric care, the case manager in the department, and a representative from the social services.

The social part of the treatment plan may comprise a description of the various social interventions that need to be carried out, such as problems concerning housing, financial support, educational activities, work, and so on.

Comments on the psychiatry plan

The municipality of Copenhagen has a Medical Advisory Group that commented on the psychiatry plan and concluded that the total number of beds in Copenhagen is too small, and should be increased by about 50. Furthermore, it was deemed important to establish differentiated housing possibilities for the most deviant and disturbed group of patients.

It is recommended that the community mental health centres each have a catchment area of 50,000–70,000 inhabitants in order to provide a more differentiated variety of treatment and a greater flexibility. The community mental health centres should not be detached from the psychiatric departments, since this may result in a lack of continuity of care for the individual patient. Furthermore, the Advisory Group sees no advantage in recruiting 'support & contact persons' attached to the social services who may be without any professional background, since this may result in a new group of helpers being involved in the treatment of psychiatric patients.

Concentrating the community psychiatric treatment on patients with severe chronic psychotic disorders has the result of leaving patients with milder disorders without any community psychiatric treatment. Consequently, the availability of community psychiatric care is at present insufficient, and it is suggested that the city of Copenhagen should increase the total number of psychiatric beds and work towards an improved access to nursing homes for psychiatric patients needing constant institutionalisation.

HOSPITAL PLAN YEAR 2000

The hospital plan of the municipality of Copenhagen (Sygehusplan H: S 2000, 1996) was completely reorganised due to a political decision to merge the three administrative bodies in charge of health services in the Copenhagen area; namely, the municipality of Copenhagen, the municipality of Frederiksberg, and the state. As a result the Copenhagen Hospital Corporation (H: S) was founded on 1 January 1995, with the aim of providing an effective use of resources, easy and equal access to all facilities provided by the health services, health service on a high professional level, continuity of care, and respect for the citizens' personal integrity.

Psychiatric services

The psychiatric services of the municipality of Copenhagen are now part of the Copenhagen Hospital Corporation. By the turn of the century the city will have five general hospitals, and each general hospital will have a psychiatric department providing comprehensive psychiatric services for the inhabitants of the catchment area. The somatic and the psychiatric part of each hospital will have similar catchment areas. Each department will have a psychiatric emergency clinic providing services around the clock for all persons who contact the clinic. All treatment is free of charge.

Each department is headed by a chief psychiatrist and a chief nurse with overall administrative and budgetary responsibility for all psychiatric services, including community mental health services. The psychiatric hospital, Skt. Hans, will remain to a large extent unchanged.

THE PRESENT STRUCTURE OF SERVICES

In 1997 the psychiatric services of the Copenhagen Hospital Corporation have the following capacity:

Kommunehospitalet*	72 beds
Bispebjerg Hospital	99 beds
Frederiksberg Hospital	96 beds
Hvidovre Hospital	120 beds
Rigshospitalet	75 beds
Skt. Hans Hospital	531 beds

*Following the establishment of the Hospital Corporation, the psychiatric departments at Kommune hospitalet will close down in the near future as the entire hospital closes down, and the department will be transferred to the new Amager Hospital that is to be established.

The mental hospital population (Skt. Hans Hospital) comprised 132

TABLE 6.1
Community Mental Health Centres in Copenhagen

Hospital	*Centre*	*Borough*
Kommunehospitalet	Indre by Amager	Indre By Christianshavn Sundby Nord Sundby Syd Amagerbro
Bispebjerg	Brønshøj Bispebjerg Ydre Nørrebro Ydre Østerbro	Brønshøj Bispebjerg Ydre Nørrebro Ydre Østerbro
Frederiksberg	Frederiksberg	Frederiksberg
Hvidovre	Valby Vanløse Vesterbro	Valby Vanløse Vesterbro Kgs. Enghave
RigsHospitalet	Møllegade Indre Østerbro	Indre Nørrebro Indre Østerbro

patients with organic brain disorders, 134 long-term patients, 114 younger patients with psychoses, 68 forensic patients and 84 patients receiving general psychiatric treatment.

Presently, the city is fully covered with community psychiatry with the community mental health centres shown in Table 6.1.

Referral to services

The referral to the emergency clinic may take place through all sorts of agencies, or by the patients themselves. No formal referral is needed and the emergency clinic has to provide acute psychiatric care to all those contacting the clinic, irrespective of their residence.

Similarly, at the community mental health centres no referral is needed, and any citizen may come and ask for psychiatric help. Services are available during normal working hours; outside working hours patients have to contact the emergency clinic.

Patients are usually referred for treatment from GPs, specialists in psychiatry or other hospital departments. More than 90% of all referrals to in-patient care are acute—and will typically follow a psychiatric assessment at the emergency clinic. The department has to accept all referrals from the catchment area.

Standard of care. Each department provides a variety of services including both open and locked wards; possibilities for day-patient care and out-patient treatment. The treatment modalities offered comprise psychopharmacological treatment, psychotherapeutic treatment, and milieu treatment as the most prevailing ones. Each department has multidisciplinary teams responsible for treatment, including psychiatrists, psychologists, social workers, physiotherapists, occupational therapists, and nurses.

The catchment area of each department is fully covered with community mental health centres. These centres are located centrally in the catchment area, which may comprise between 25,000–90,000 inhabitants.

Liaison psychiatric services

At all the general hospitals an extensive liaison psychiatric service takes place. Typically one or more specialists in psychiatry focuses on this task and carries out psychiatric consultation to the different departments. Regular conferences may take place with, for example, child psychiatric units, pain clinics, neurological units, burns units or other specialities needing frequent psychiatric expertise.

Community mental health service

Each community mental health clinic has a multidisciplinary team headed by a psychiatric consultant and a chief nurse, with the same professional groups as in the hospital department, and is under the administrative responsibility of the department. The community clinic typically provides out-patient care, to some extent day-care, and carries out assessment interviews for referrals from the catchment area. Typically, the community clinic may offer extensive out-going services with home visits, working with the social support system and closely collaborating with primary health care and social services. There is a close collaboration between the community clinic and the in-patient department with various kinds of joint patient conferences, educational programmes, rotation of staff, etc. On an individual patient basis, staff members collaborate in relation to case management to ensure optimum continuity of care.

Forensic services

As all departments have comprehensive responsibility, they receive forensic patients, transferred from prisons, police stations, etc., or patients having a sentence with a psychiatric condition. The psychiatric hospital has a special ward for forensic care, primarily for psychiatrically sentenced patients needing long-term admission. It has recently been concluded that in order to solve the present problems with the increasing number of forensic patients, an increase in the bed capacity for this patient population is required. It is recommended that forensic psychiatry is primarily concentrated in the psychiatric hospital, where further locked wards should be established.

Patients with problems of abuse

Alcohol abuse. Alcohol represents a major problem in the city of Copenhagen. Previously, patients with alcohol problems were frequently admitted to psychiatric departments. Over the last decade, a significant decrease in the number of admissions with alcohol-related disorders has been observed. This is partly due to the fact that the emergency clinics at the psychiatric departments in Copenhagen provide treatment for withdrawal symptoms without admitting the patient. Only a small proportion of patients showing psychotic symptoms or very disturbed behaviour will be admitted to psychiatric departments. Patients with alcohol problems, who do not require admission, may receive treatment in various settings. Related to all hospitals are alcohol clinics with interdisciplinary teams which provide medical and social help to patients with alcohol disorders.

A large number of other clinics exist using different treatment models. Among these the following could be mentioned: Alcoholics Anonymous, Blue Cross, Minnesota model, and several types of private clinics. There is very limited collaboration between the different agencies providing care for patients with alcohol problems. This makes it difficult to get an overall view of the size of the problem and an evaluation of the services provided.

Drug abuse. The treatment of drug addicts has traditionally been placed outside the health services. In Copenhagen the social services have established a number of local district centres to take care of this population. Generally, patients with substance abuse will get in contact with psychiatric services if they have a dual diagnosis of substance abuse and a psychotic disorder, or if they manifest suicidal behaviour.

Initiatives according to the hospital plan

It is specifically mentioned in the plan (Sygehusplan H:S 2000, 1996) that psychiatry will receive top priority. Among the necessary initiatives to take place are the following:

1. The present capacity of psychiatric beds is inadequate and increased resources have to be allocated to psychiatry.
2. The number of psychiatric beds in acute and general psychiatry will be increased by about 50 beds.
3. Community mental health care will be further expanded and the whole Copenhagen area will be covered with community psychiatric care.
4. Catchment areas of somatic and psychiatric departments will be identical.
5. The facilities for the psychiatric departments will be improved. This implies that any department establishing new beds will provide single room facilities for all patients, and departments already established will be transformed into single bed units by the year 2002.
6. A limited number of rooms providing two bedroom units will still exist to satisfy a specific wish for some patients.

PROVISION AND UTILISATION OF PSYCHIATRIC SERVICES

Provision of beds

In 1976, Denmark had approximately 2.4 psychiatric beds per 1000 inhabitants. In total, the number of psychiatric beds amounted to about 10,000. In 1987 about 2600 beds were adminstratively transferred to social services, as they were placed in gerontopsychiatric nursing hospitals that were taken over by the social services. Consequently, the number of beds decreased from the 2.4 per 1000 to 1.2 per 1000 in 1987.

The Ministry of Health and the Ministry of Social Affairs (1993) reported that the development of beds per 1000 inhabitants in Denmark during the period 1989–1993 decreased from 1.0 to 0.8 per 1000 inhabitants. Since then, the total number of beds has decreased by a further 5% to the present (1995) figure of 4065 beds in all psychiatric institutions.

The number of psychiatric beds per 1000 inhabitants in Copenhagen reached a peak in the late 1970s, when Copenhagen had about 7 psychiatric beds per 1000 inhabitants. However, at that time the city also partly provided mental health care for the municipality of Frederiksberg and a neighbouring county. Due to the administrative change in 1987 the number of psychiatric beds in the city was reduced to 3.1 psychiatric beds per 1000 inhabitants.

In the municipality of Copenhagen the number of beds in 1989–1993 decreased from 2.3 to 1.8 per 1000 inhabitants, and in the municipality of Frederiksberg (now part of the Copenhagen Hospital Corporation) the number of beds increased from 1.0 to 1.1 per 1000 inhabitants. At the establishment of Copenhagen Hospital Corporation, the number of beds was approximately 1.7 per 1000.

Utilisation of services

Concomitantly with the reduction in the number of beds we have experienced a reduction in the number of long-stay patients. Furthermore, we have observed that the average number of days per admission in Denmark declined from 48 in 1989 to 40 in 1992. During the same period the annual number of admissions did not decline but remained relatively constant at around 35,000—but with a change in the diagnostic distribution, as the number of admissions of schizophrenic patients has increased, whereas a decrease has been observed in the admission of patients with neurotic disorders.

In the municipality of Copenhagen the average length of stay fell from 71 days in 1989 to 39 days in 1993.

According to the Danish National Psychiatric Case Register all Danish psychiatric departments had 34,248 admissions (17,148 males and 17,100 females) and 33,912 discharges in 1995 (16,991 males and 16,921 females). Out of these, 4895 (2529 males and 2366 females) were admitted and 5936 (3070 males and 2866 females) were discharged from all the psychiatric departments in the municipality of Copenhagen. Further, 1593 (1050 males and 543 females) were admitted and 1606 (1054 males and 552 females) patients were discharged from the psychiatric hospital Skt. Hans. Whereas the country as a whole, and the acute departments in Copenhagen, observed almost similar numbers of male and female admissions and discharges, males comprised 66% of both admissions and discharges from the psychiatric hospital. This male preponderance was particularly pronounced at the forensic ward and the ward for patients with various kinds of abuse.

The consumption of hospital days in Copenhagen has been more than halved during the period 1970–84. The reduction in hospital days is found in all age groups, but in particular among the middle-aged and elderly. Further, psychiatric patients up to the age of 45 in 1984 consumed about 50% of the total number of hospital days, and over the years this age group in absolute numbers has had a rather constant consumption of hospital days (Direktoratet for Københavns Hospitalsvaesen, 1987).

Copenhagen had in the same period experienced a reduction in the population by 23%. In the light of this, it was stated in the psychiatry plan that the steep reduction in psychiatric bed days for the middle-aged and elderly was due to a combination of demographic factors, the increased emphasis on out-patient treatment and day hospital treatment, together with the fact that a number of these patients (in particular those with organic brain disorder) had been transferred to the social services.

The reduction in bed day consumption for the younger age group was related to an altered treatment ideology, which placed emphasis on out-patient treatment and short-term in-patient episodes.

With a regard to diagnostic groups, the reduction in hospital days is found in all the main diagnostic groups, but particularly organic disorders and reactive disorders (including personality disorders), alcohol and substance abuse and neurotic disorders, while the two largest diagnostic groups with regard to consumption of hospital beds are now, as previously, people with schizophrenia and with reactive disorders.

Out-patient care, on the other hand, has increased in Denmark, where 53,544 (23,045 males and 30,499 females) started day- or out-patient treatment in 1995. In Copenhagen, 7410 (3586 males and 3824 females) started day- or out-patient treatment in 1995. Of these, 1414 (717 males and 697 females) started treatment in the community mental health clinics, which corresponds to 26% of all day- or out-patient treatment started at the psychiatric departments in Copenhagen. Community psychiatric services are now available for about 80% of the Danish population, but with regional variations from 20% to 100%.

The Psychiatry Plan concluded that the demographic development, the development in treatment methods, the change towards increased day hospitals and extramural activity and the establishment of community mental health centres could be expected to reduce further the need for psychiatric hospital beds in the years to come. Further, it also concluded that a reduction is likely to be seen in the use of psychiatric beds even for the younger age groups.

Staff

Based on figures from the largest (1997) psychiatric department in Copenhagen (Hvidovre Hospital), the staff related to psychiatry in 1997 was calculated showing per 1000 inhabitants:

0.3	doctors
0.09	psychologists
0.1	social workers
0.06	physiotherapists
0.1	occupational therapists
1.0	psychiatric nurses
0.6	mental health assistants and other aides.

Of these: 0.08 doctors, 0.03 psychologists, 0.04 social workers, 0.02 physiotherapists, 0.05 occupational therapists, 0.1 psychiatric nurses, and 0.01 mental health assistants and other aides worked in community mental health settings. Nursing staff are thus relatively less commonly working in community mental health compared in particular to social workers, occupational therapists and psychologists.

The number of staff in Copenhagen related to community psychiatry differed from the country as a whole. Denmark had 0.04 doctors per 1000 inhabitants, 0.04 nurses and a total of 0.16 staff members per 1000 inhabitants working in community mental health settings.

Physical facilities for psychiatric care

In 1996, the Ministry of Health (Sundhedsministeriet, 1997) carried out a questionnaire regarding the physical facilities at the various psychiatric departments in Denmark, as a consequence of the agreement between the government and the regional health authorities to allocate increased resources to mental health, and in particular to improve the physical facilities of the various psychiatric institutions. The survey showed for Copenhagen an average of 14 beds per ward. Of all beds 48% were located on open wards, 19% on locked wards, 12% in long-term care, 7% in forensic care, and 5% in gerontopsychiatric units. Single rooms were found among 30% of all beds, ranging from 20% in the open wards to 59% in long-term wards; 49% of all beds were located in rooms with two beds and the remaining 21% in rooms with more than two beds.

Copenhagen had relatively fewer single rooms, as the whole country had

42% of beds located in single rooms, 45% in two-bed rooms and only 12% in rooms with more than two beds. The number of available toilets and bathrooms were calculated and showed that each ward in Copenhagen had on average 2.4 toilets, 1.0 bathrooms and 1.6 combined toilet/bath. Less than 1% of the rooms had their own toilet or bath. The availability of sanitary facilities did not differ from the country as a whole.

The availability of other types of facilities was analysed, showing that in Copenhagen 79% of all wards provided the patients with a sitting room, 90% with dining facilities, 21% with separate rooms for smokers and 33% with non-smoking facilities. Music or TV rooms were available in 20% of the cases, and visiting areas in 30%. Here again no difference was observed with regard to these facilities from the country as a whole. In Copenhagen access to outdoor facilities was available in 49% of the wards. In 41% of the cases the wards could only provide non-secure outdoor facilities, and in 26% the department could provide secured outdoor facilities. In the country as a whole 83% of all wards had some kind of availability of outdoor facilities. Thus, we see that Copenhagen differs significantly with respect to this. The vast majority (78%) of the departments in Copenhagen were located in buildings dated back before 1950. However, only 10% of them had not undergone any reconstructions. It is characteristic that all locked departments had undergone some kind of reconstruction since 1950.

Access to various therapeutic facilities was highly prevalent. In Copenhagen, 90% of wards had access to physiotherapy and gymnastics, 93% to occupational therapy, 90% to kitchen training and 86% to various kinds of workshops. Compared to the country as a whole there was easier access to all facilities in the Copenhagen area.

Free hospital choice

According to Danish legislation, citizens have a free choice with regard to basic hospital care. This implies that psychiatric patients may ask to be treated at any psychiatric department, according to their choice, and that the department cannot refuse to provide services free of charge. In practice it has, however, turned out that this right has not been used by many citizens, and that at any given time only a few percent of the admissions in Copenhagen are due to a specific request to be treated at a given department, whereas the vast majority get treated at their regional psychiatric department.

ROLE OF USERS AND RELATIVES

Several organisations exist in Denmark which represent the interests of users and relatives. It is characteristic that these organisations have been able to lobby effectively for the rights and influence of users and relatives.

These organisations have developed alternative models for the provision of psychiatric care, and have been successful in obtaining political contacts. The relation between these consumer organisations and institutional psychiatric care is to a large extent based on personal contacts and less on formalized collaboration.

In Copenhagen, however, a number of psychiatric departments have established relative groups, psycho-educational groups, open counselling, and so on. In the community mental health centres there is a formalised collaboration, as each centre has a consumer council with representatives from users, relatives and staff, who together discuss issues such as the various activities offered, and the facilities available. According to the Danish Mental Health Act it is also mandatory for psychiatric departments to have open patient meetings on a regular basis between the head of the department and patients admitted, to discuss the quality of services, availability of therapy and activities, etc.

There is an increasing recognition among professionals that the influence and feedback from consumers has been insufficient up until now, and that psychiatric services could benefit from an increasing influence from such groups.

FUTURE CHALLENGES

We are presently witnessing different developments in the organisation of mental health services.

In some regions of Denmark, out-patient and community psychiatric care have been taken over by social services, with a consequent decrease in the medical impact, whereas other regions—among them Copenhagen—have established community psychiatric services with a clear medical responsibility.

Psychiatrists generally agree that the key population for psychiatric care is the chronic psychotic population. As a consequence, large groups of patients with less severe disorders (e.g. milder depressions, traumatic reactions, stress-related disorders) are treated outside institutional psychiatric care, frequently by GPs or psychologists. Other groups, e.g. patients with problems of abuse, are receiving treatment at special institutions. If this development continues further, we may end up having psychiatrists with a highly specialised, but rather narrow, expertise. It is questionable whether this is beneficial for the profession in the long run.

We are experiencing in some areas a movement towards demedicalisation of psychiatric care. The same deprofessionalisation is seen where psychiatry has been administratively transferred to the social sector, thereby removing the psychiatric discipline from other medical disciplines—a development towards which the Danish Psychiatric Association has been critical.

Related hereto, we experience a layman's wish for deprofessionalisation and an interest among paramedical groups in the less severe disorders.

One way to fight this development, and join forces instead, could be to allow the consumers of services greater impact, and draw upon their experiences in the professional work.

The city of Copenhagen has avoided this development. It has constantly worked on the principle that psychiatry is a medical discipline, and that psychiatric services are an integral part of the general medical services, with clear responsibility to provide the best therapy available consistent with accepted scientific knowledge and ethical principles, and to carry out research and evaluation in order to improve the quality of care and availibility of the most up-to-date treatment to the citizens.

REFERENCES

Direktoratet for Københavns Hospitalsvæsen (Directorate Copenhagen Health Services). (1987). *Forslag til psykiatriplan for Københavns Kommune 1988–2000. (Proposal for a psychiatry plan for the municipality of Copenhagen 1988–2000.)* Copenhagen: Direktoratet.

Knudsen, H.C., Jessen-Petersen, B., Klitgaard, V., Krasnik, A., Nordentoft, M., & Sælan, H. (1992). *Distriktspsykiatri i København. En evaluering af de første to år. (Community psychiatry in Copenhagen. An evaluation after the first two years).* Copenhagen: Institute of Social Medicine, Copenhagen University.

Statistical Yearbook for the Copenhagen Region. (1995). Copenhagen: Municipality of Copenhagen.

Sundhedsdirektoratet (The health directorate). (1993). *Psychiatry plan for the municipality of Copenhagen.* Copenhagen: Sundhedsdirektoratet.

Sundhedsministeriet (Ministry of Health). (1997). *De fysiske rammer på de psykiatriske afdelinger i Danmark. (The physical conditions of the Danish psychiatric departments).* Copenhagen: Sundhedsministeriet.

Sundhedsministeriet & Socialministeriet (Ministry of Health, Ministry Social Affairs). (1993). *Fremrykning af indsatsen for sindslidende.* Copenhagen: Sundhedsministeriet & Sundhedsministeriet.

Sygehusplan H: S 2000 (Hospitalplan Copenhagen Hospital Corporation Year 2000). (1996). Copenhagen: Hovedstadens Sygehusfællesskab.

CHAPTER SEVEN

Mental health in the city of Kobe, Japan

Naotaka Shinfuku
Kobe University School of Medicine, Japan
Susumu Sugawara and Teruo Yanaka
Yadokari-no-sato, Oomiya-city, Japan
Mariko Kimura
Tokai University, Japan

THE CITY OF KOBE, JAPAN

Population and other general outlines

Kobe city is situated in the Kansai area, close to Osaka and Kyoto. It is the prefectural capital of Hyogo Prefecture (population: 5.5 million) and with a population of 1.5 million, is ranked as the sixth largest city in Japan. Kobe city was one of two ports opened for foreigners after the Meiji Revolution which took place about 130 years ago, and was subsequently developed as a major port in western Japan. Because of this historical background, the city is famous for active international relations. Several heavy industries, including ship building, are located in the city. The city is served by Shinkansen, national railways, several private transport lines, and access to the airports is easy. Kobe and its surrounding cities host a number of prestigious national and private universities and colleges. Kobe University is the major academic institution in the area, with 11 schools and several research centres. The International Centre for Medical Research (ICMR) was established in 1979 at Kobe University School of Medicine to promote collaboration in medical sciences with southeast Asian countries, and the WHO Kobe Centre was established in 1996. In short, Kobe city is one of the most attractive cities in Japan and rated as the most desirable city to live in. It is also the favourite place for domestic tourism, particularly among young women, due to its international flavour and its modern shopping arcades.

Health indicators

Health indicators in Kobe are similar to the average in Japan. The infant mortality rate in Japan is 4.2 per 1000 births, which is the lowest in the world. The average length of life is 80–83 for women and 76 for men. Hyogo Prefecture is a relatively wealthy prefecture and the percentage of the population receiving the Life Protection scheme from the government (a measurement of poverty) is low. The homeless are almost non-existent in Kobe, and street children are unseen. Amphetamine abuse among members of a criminal syndicate (yakuza) and the abuse of stimulants among young school drop-outs are reported by the mass media. However, the extent of these problems is small compared to their magnitude in the USA and in European countries.

Kobe city has a relatively large foreign population (more than 1% of the total population) compared to other cities in Japan. A considerable number of traders from China, Europe, India and Korea settled in Kobe over the past 100 years. Recently, resettlement of refugees from Vietnam started in the suburbs of the city.

The great Hanshin Awaji earthquake

Kobe city was an epicentre of the Hanshin Awaji earthquake which devastated Hanshin Awaji area on the morning of 17 January 1995. The earthquake killed more than 6300 people and injured more than 40,000. Almost 247,000 houses were destroyed. More than 310,000 people lost their houses and had to stay in shelters. At present, almost 20,000 people are still staying in temporary houses built for victims. Kobe city lost almost 100,000 members of the population after the earthquake as a result of emigration to nearby cities which were unaffected by the disaster. Unemployment, economic difficulties, and long-term health consequences are placing an enormous burden on the affected vulnerable population, such as the elderly and handicapped.

MENTAL HEALTH SERVICES IN KOBE

In Japan, the number of psychiatric beds increased tremendously in the 1960s due to the government policy of stimulating the building of psychiatric hospitals by the private sector. The number of psychiatric beds was 95,067 in 1960, and increased to 172,950 in 1965, 247,725 in 1970 and 268,669 in 1973. The rate of increase between 1973 and 1993 was more gradual, with the number of beds rising to a maximum in 1993 of 362,963. In 1994, the number decreased for the first time since the Second World War, to 362,235. This reduction was related to the gradual shifting of national mental health policy towards community care. At present, almost 90% of psychiatric beds are located in about 1000 private psychiatric hospitals scattered all over Japan, each with average bed numbers of between 200-400.

Although they are private psychiatric hospitals, fees for treatment (both in-patient and out-patients) are covered by national health insurance schemes. Therefore, private hospitals have been rather keen to keep as many patients as possible as long as possible for financial reasons. This system has resulted in a very long average length of stay of mental patients in Japan.

Budget for mental health services

In Japan, the majority of health expenditure is covered by national health insurance schemes. Therefore, it is hard to identify the exact amount spent for mental health services. In the 1997 financial year, Hyogo Prefecture (5.5 million population) will spend $30 million on mental health and welfare services, out of its total health budget of $330 million,. This means that about 9% of the health budget of the local government will be spent on various programmes and activities related to mental health and welfare services. However, this does not include medical fees for the majority of in-patients. These fees are mostly covered by national insurance schemes or by the Government Life Protection scheme (for the poor). Kobe city has no separate mental health policy and programme. The mental health policy and programme of Kobe city constitutes a part of the mental health policy and programme of Hyogo Prefectural Government in general. National mental health policy is decided by the Division of Mental Health at the Ministry of Health and Welfare in Tokyo, and the mental health policy of Kobe city is in turn decided by the Mental Health Section of the Department of Health at Hyogo Prefectural Government. The first author is a member of the Advisory Board of Hyogo Prefectural Mental Health Committee.

Main features of the mental health services

Different kinds of facilities and manpower comprise mental health services in Kobe city. Psychiatric hospitals and psychiatric clinics are major sources for the treatment and care of mental patients. There have been a growing number of private psychiatric clinics. The Prefectural Mental Health Centre at Kobe city focuses on promotion, prevention and education for health workers. It also organises day care services, and provides consultation services for patients. Local health centres are increasingly engaged in consultation and community services for mental patients. The government is currently promoting the establishment of different kinds of community programmes for chronic patients and elderly patients.

Different service providers

Psychiatric Hospitals. In 1996, there were 42 psychiatric hospitals at Hyogo Prefecture. The total number of beds was 12,201. These hospitals are categorised as follows:

Psychiatric beds at two university hospitals	60 beds
Two prefectural mental hospitals	605 beds
Psychiatric beds at municipal hospitals	100 beds
Twenty-eight Private psychiatric hospital foundations	8933 beds
Nine privately owned psychiatric hospitals	2503 beds

In Japan, psychiatric hospitals have by far the largest resources in psychiatric manpower. Even a majority of community mental health programmes are supported by staff members of psychiatric hospitals.

Table 7.1 shows the number of psychiatric hospital beds in Hyogo Prefecture. There has been a decrease of psychiatric beds since 1995, due to the Awaji Hanshin earthquake.

Psychiatric hospitals deal with patients with behavioural and emotional symptoms. Compulsory admission based on the Mental Health and Welfare Law is one of the major responsibilities of psychiatric hospitals. Public funds are provided for: the treatment of patients; hospitalisation under the medical protection scheme; and the compulsory hospitalisation scheme. Local government support services relate to emergency psychiatric care.

TABLE 7.1
Changes in Number of Psychiatric Hospitals and Psychiatric In-patients in Hyogo Prefecture

Year		*Number of hospital*	*Number of beds*	*Beds per 10,000 pop.*	*Number of In-patients*	*Patients Hospitalised by Court Order*
1994	Hyogo Pref.	42	12,152	22.1	11,830	227
	Japan	1672	362,235	29.0	343,126	6408
1995	Hyogo Pref.	40	12,201	22.1	11,912	228
	Japan	1671	362,180	29.0	340,785	5905
1996	Hyogo Pref.*	30	8367	21.0	8110	172
	Japan	1667	361,053	18.8	339,762	5436

* 1996 decrease is due to the Awaji Hanshin Earthquake.

They collaborate with psychiatric hospitals in the community to develop rotational responsibilities for emergency care on holidays and at night time.

Psychiatric clinics

The number of specialist psychiatric clinics is rather small—about 1000 in the whole of Japan, and 92 in Hyogo Prefecture. However, the official number of psychiatric clinics in Japan is around 2600, a figure which includes clinics run by internists and neurologists, who are permitted to treat mental patients. Although the number of clinics is small at present, this is the category of mental health service with the fastest growth-rate in Japan.

Psychiatric beds in general hospitals

Kobe University Hospital has a small number of psychiatric beds, and is used as a teaching hospital for medical students and post-graduate students. In Japan, very few general hospitals have psychiatric wards. However, an increasing number of general hospitals employ psychiatrists for liaison services, particularly for terminal cases.

Mental health centres

The Hyogo Prefectural Mental Health Centre was established in Kobe city in 1968, and plays a key role in mental health in terms of promotion, prevention and rehabilitation. It is also expected to provide technical guidance and support for mental health activities carried out at other health centres. In Japan, mental health centres were established in 1960 and 1980 in each of the 46 prefectures. Hyogo Prefectural Mental Health Centre played a coordinating role in the provision of mental health care for victims of the great Hanshin Awaji earthquake.

Health centres

Based on the guidelines of the Mental Health and Welfare Law and the Community Health Law, health centres (of which there are 852 in Japan, each having a catchment area of around 100,000–200,000 people) have been requested to play a coordinating role in the provision of mental health activities carried out in the community. Health centres used to focus their activities on the MCH (Mother and Child Health) and anti-TB programme, but changed their focus recently to concentrate on geriatric and mental health services.

Community programmes

In 1996, there were 98 occupational training centres, 33 short stay facilities, 79 welfare homes, 91 community vocational training facilities, 11 residential vocational training facilities, 3 welfare factories and 22 community living support programmes, all for people with mental illness throughout Japan. Yadokarino-sato is one of the pioneers of community living support programmes for mentally ill people (see 'Mental health and welfare programmes in general hospitals', below).

Several of the above-listed community programmes operate in Kobe and other parts of Hyogo Prefecture. The government is planning both to increase the number and to promote the quality of these community programmes as part of a National Master Plan for Disabled Persons enacted in 1995.

Payment

Table 7.2 shows the different payment schemes for mental health services at Hyogo Prefecture. Public funds contribute the major part. National insurance schemes account for 60% of public funding based on mental health law (involuntary hospitalisation), life protection schemes, geriatric protection schemes and child protection schemes contribute another 40%. Very few people pay privately for psychiatric services.

The total budget for the mental health programme of Hyogo Prefectural Government is 3 billion yen (equivalent to approximately US $29 million). The majority of these funds are used to cover the treatment of patients admitted on medical protection schemes and involuntary hospitalisation

TABLE 7.2

	Changes in in-patient population (by financial support)		
Type of financial support	*1994*	*1995*	*1996*
Mental health law	227	224	156
Life protection law	2563	2466	1519
Others (Geriatric protection law, etc.)	2539	2540	2202
National insurance	6466	6224	3864
Private	3	1	0
Others	32	37	123
Total	11,830	11,472	7864

* 1996 decrease is due to the Hanshin Awaji earthquake.

schemes. These schemes are not covered by usual national insurance schemes or by life protection schemes for the poor.

According to the report from the Hyogo Prefectural local government, the 3021 million yen will be used to support the following mental health and welfare activities for 1997:

1. Community mental health and welfare programme 34M ¥
2. Rehabilitation of mental patients 297M ¥
3. Geriatric mental health and welfare services including medical cost subsidy for patients under geriatric medical schemes. Without medical cost subsidy, the budget for the programme is 19M ¥. 1279M ¥
4. Psychiatric in-patients treatment services including cost subsidy for medical protection and involuntary treatment 1411M ¥

Mental health activities used to be grouped under these four major headings, but after the Hanshin Awaji earthquake, a new programme of psychological care for the victims of disaster was added.

Patients

Table 7.3 shows the distribution of psychiatric in-patients in Hyogo Prefecture by diagnostic category. Schizophrenia accounts for more than 60% of in-patients. However, the number of geriatric in-patients has increased gradually.

TABLE 7.3
Psychiatric In-patients in Hyogo Prefecture by Diagnostic Category

	Changes in in-patient population (by diagnostic criteria)		
Diagnostic Category	*1994*	*1995*	*1996*
Schizophrenia	6929	6823	4775
Depression, mood disorder	614	558	329
Epilepsy	297	287	199
Geriatric Mental Disorder	1872	1709	1251
Alcohol & substance abuse	630	608	298
Others	1488	1109	1258
Total	11,830	11,094	8110

* 1996 decrease is due to the Hanshin Awaji earthquake.

Staff

The number of psychiatrists in Japan in 1994 was around 9512, or 4.3% of all medical doctors. The precise number of psychiatric nurses is not known. However, it is estimated that around 10% of all nurses are working in mental health services (around 80-90,000 nurses out of a national total of 862,013). In Japan, almost 20% (18.7%) of all hospital beds are psychiatric beds. Hospital services require a lot of nursing manpower. Occupational therapists are often in high demand, as their number is relatively small in Japan (7708 in 1994). As there is no specialist certificate for psychiatrists in Japan, no figures are available for numbers of staff or trainee psychiatrists. Also, there are very few posts available for psychologists in psychiatric services. The number of psychologists working in day-care services is increasing.

The demarcation of roles between hospital nurses, community nurses, and public health nurses has little meaning in Japan. Community mental health services, such as visits to people in their homes, are carried out by hospital nurses in many cases. Also, public health nurses in the 852 public health centres (Hokensyo) in Japan are increasingly engaged in community mental health services, as their traditional activities such as vaccination and work on the anti-tuberculosis programme have markedly decreased. Social workers and psychiatric social workers are not well established in Japan. The number of such staff operating in psychiatric services is still very small. The overall staffing figures per 100,000 people are as follows:

Medical doctors (all)	176
Psychiatrists	7.6
Nurses (all)	689
Mental health nurses	60–70
Occupational therapists	6.2

The required number of medical staff working at medical institutions is determined by Japanese medical law. In psychiatric hospitals, the number of doctors and nurses can be reduced according to the nature of the care involved. In psychiatric hospitals, a minimum staffing level of three doctors is required per 156 beds, compared to 52 beds in a general hospital. One additional doctor is required for every increase of 48 patients in a psychiatric hospital, while in a general hospital one additional doctor is required for every increase of 6 patients. A similar situation applies regarding the number of nurses. One nurse is required for every addition of 6 patients in a psychiatric hospital, compared with one nurse for every 4 additional patients in a general hospital. In Japan in

1994, an average of 2.5 doctors and 24.0 nurses per 100 beds were working in psychiatric hospitals, compared with 10.8 doctors and 42.7 nurses in general hospitals.

Coordination

The overall programme is coordinated by the Mental Health Division of the Hyogo Prefectural Government, which is linked in with various mental health resources in Hyogo Prefecture, as well as with general health care services. Health and social services are well integrated, especially for geriatric mental health services. The Mental health centre has a close working relationship with schools. Private and public psychiatric hospitals are obliged to work closely with the police for cases of involuntary hospitalisation. A combination of private and public services is available in the community for mental patients, as well as for the general population. In a unique way, this system seems fairly comprehensive and covers almost all the needs of the population of Hyogo Prefecture.

SOME RECENT POSITIVE FEATURES OF MENTAL HEALTH SERVICES IN KOBE

Increase of private psychiatric clinics

One important recent development is the modification of national insurance schemes so that they favour care in the community. This has stimulated the opening of private psychiatric clinics in major cities. In Hyogo Prefecture, there are at present 92 private psychiatric clinics. These clinics began to be opened in the 1960s, and have gradually increased in number. Young psychiatrists interested in community care joined forces to open psychiatric clinics. Also, in the 1990s, the government set a limit on the number of beds, including psychiatric beds, for each geographic medical service area. This has prevented psychiatric hospitals from increasing their bed capacity. The opening of new hospitals has become almost impossible. This situation has favoured the opening of many psychiatric out-patient clinics in the community.

At present, the number of psychiatric clinics in Japan is around 1000—almost the same as the number of psychiatric hospitals. Private psychiatric clinics usually receive between 60 and 100 patients a day. Almost all patients are covered by national insurance schemes. Day care services are attached to some private psychiatric clinics. The image of private psychiatric clinics in the USA and in Europe, which portrays them as treating only the very rich using psychoanalysis, is very far removed from the private psychiatric clinic in Japan. The increase of private psychiatric clinics will surely be the most important feature in the development of community-based mental health services in Japan.

Yadokarinosato: Its philosophy, value, and practice

History

Yadokarinosato (literally 'a home for hermit crabs'), was a project born out of social work in a private psychiatric hospital. In the late 1960s, Teruo Yanaka, president of Yadokarinosato, was working as a social worker in a private mental hospital, engaged in the rehabilitation of in-patients in Saitama Prefecture. At that time, and even now, it is often the case that patients stay hospitalised for extended periods in Japan, compared to the average hospital stay in developed countries. This is due to a scarcity both of community support services, and of family members who can accept them at home. In 1970, Yanaka found a place for discharged patients to live upstairs in a factory, with the aim of turning it into a transitional house where discharged in-patients were sent to work for sheltered employment. However, this idea failed to gain approval, as the hospital authorities argued that they might be blamed in the case of any accidents. In spite of this rejection by the hospital, and in addition to his work at the hospital, Yanaka rented the place for these patients to live, and began a housing programme. This was the beginning of Yadokarinosato.

When the hospital discontinued its day-care programme, it was assimilated as part of the programme at Yadokarinosato and make it into a social club. During this period, staff lived with members, and provided support in preparing meals, life-skills training and finding sheltered employment. Later, this half-way house was closed due to the fear that it might create another institution. The focus of support then shifted to securing apartments, providing support in finding jobs in market employment, creating an environment for members to develop their own support networks among people with psychiatric disabilities, and organising a club for mental health consumers.

At present, Yadokarinosato has been approved as a corporate juridical body by Saitama Prefecture. As of February 1996, it holds 114 people with psychiatric disabilities. There are 26 full-time staff, including 16 social workers with the Bachelor of Social Work, one psychologist with the Bachelor of Psychology, several management staff, and 11 part-time staff. Programmes provided by Yadokarinosato are described as follows: There are four sites called Support Centres in the southern part of Omiya city, each with a group home and a sheltered workshop. Each site also has three to four staff (sometimes just one), who are there to provide support services and case management. At one of these support centres, there is a meal preparation and delivery section. Meals are delivered to group homes and apartments of the members. There is a hostel near the head office which provides short-stay, respite care, and transitional living services. The head office is responsible for the management and development of apartments. Recently, a new building was opened to set up a printing factory, and a public relations office. Yadokarinosato also provides staff training programmes for community mental health professionals.

Philosophy

It was Yanaka's idea to create a place for people with psychiatric disabilities separate from the mental hospital, where members could feel a sense of belonging. The role of the staff is to provide support to complement the abilities and skills which have been lost as a result of mental illness and long-term hospitalisation. People with psychiatric disabilities require various kinds of support in order to live in the community. The focus of rehabilitation should be on the creation of various kinds of support around such people in order to make community living possible, rather than on the eradication of symptoms. In the process of building support around members, Yadokarinosato has demonstrated the importance of psychosocial aspects of support in the community, which have been different from those provided in psychiatric hospitals.

Providing support so that they can live just like anybody else in the community. It has been a service goal for Yadokarinosato to 'allow persons with psychiatric disabilities to live an ordinary life'. Yadokarinosato has accumulated data from practice in the community, and turned it both into written materials which describe the difficulties of community living, and programmes which require further development by mental health professionals in Japan. This has formed part of the education of professionals, government officials and even physicians in the mental health field. The accumulated knowledge and methodology developed through practice in the community has provided a basis from which new principles of social rehabilitation and mental health policy can be formed. It has influenced policy makers in the mental health services in Japan to shift the focus of rehabilitation and funding away from the hospital-based medical model to a community-based model, since the reforms of the Japanese Mental Health Act in 1987, when an article of social rehabilitation was added to the Act, and public funding increasingly began to be put into small-scale community programmes. In this sense, the Act addressed the importance of the well-being of persons with psychiatric disabilities and the provision of support needed to realise community living, while the previous act addressed security and protection measures of the community from the mentally ill.

Providing a support for daily living. Providing support for daily living is a way to normalise the lives of persons with psychiatric disabilities. Providing support includes building support networks and communication between persons with psychiatric disabilities themselves, as well as the provision of support in areas such as management of medication, housing, and participation with other social activities in the community. Yadokarinosato also emphasised that it is important to obtain agreement between a consumer and a physician on the issue of medication: allowing a person sufficient medication to facilitate living in the community with some symptoms remaining; as opposed to being prescribed a dosage that renders the person dysfunctional, or concentrating efforts solely on the eradication of symptoms.

Yadokarinosato also presents a new concept of life for persons with psychiatric disabilities. Among rehabilitation professionals, social skills training was considered necessary for persons with psychiatric disabilities, and the goal is to allow such people to return to work in the open employment market. This goes against the traditional goal of rehabilitation for persons with psychiatric illness. Yadokarinosato introduced a new concept of social participation. This was to develop networks among persons with psychiatric disabilities, to enable them to feel empowered by sharing similar experiences of mental illness and hospitalisation. This gives a new meaning to the lives of persons with psychiatric disabilities, and expands the horizons and the definition of rehabilitation for them.

At Yadokarinosato, the goal for providing support is 'living just like anybody else'. The concept of 'living just like anybody else' attunes to the concept of normalisation, and provides guidelines for how the professionals treat people with psychiatric disabilities. Firstly, people with psychiatric disabilities should be treated as ordinary people living in the community, rather than as a person with a psychiatric illness, regardless of their disability. In other words, 'the person should be first, and the disability second'. Secondly, we deal with a person who is responsible for their actions just like anybody else, regardless of psychiatric disabilities. In this sense, we ask a person to take responsibility for their actions, and we respect the person's decision. Thirdly, people have the right to have their community living secured, and necessary support should be provided to make life in the community possible. Fourthly, leading an ordinary life in the community means respecting one's own decision to choose one's lifestyle, rather than having a mental health professional force a ready-made programme on the person. By forcing a ready-made programme (such as skills training), there is a danger of assimilating people with disabilities into one mode of training. While each has their own wish, and their own disabilities, the support required may differ. It is more humane to have an individualised programme, creating one if necessary; and, sometimes, the support has to be tailored to individual needs.

Methodology of providing support for daily living. Comparisons between the traditional medical model and the life model, upon which Yadokarinosato's programme is based, have been made in various aspects of treatment (Table 7.4).

Under the life model concept, six subconcepts have been used to describe ways of helping:

1. If there is a sufficient variety of programmes from which to choose, consumers can develop a sense of how to make their own decisions, based on the information provided by the staff.
2. Consumers decide which lifestyle they wish to adopt. The identification of support needed, decisions, and solutions to problems, are all conducted by the consumer through discussion with staff. This is contrary to the traditional ladders model of rehabilitation training.
3. The life model allows a person with psychiatric disabilities to live just like anybody else in the community. By providing support for daily living, the focus is not on guidance or training, but on creating services and programmes which allow people to be themselves
4. Everybody has their own will, even though they might not be manifesting a strong motivation as a result of exhaustion from illness.

TABLE 7.4
Comparison between the Medical Model and the Life Model

	Traditional Social Rehabilitation (Medical Model)	*Providing Support in Daily Living (Life Model)*
Decision maker	Helper (professional)	Consumer
Responsibility	Health care professional	Decision by the consumer
Intervention	Help to lead regulated life	Help to allow the consumer to make their own decisions
Focus of treatment	Diagnosis and symptoms	Identifying areas where support is needed
Relationship	Treatment, helper and helpee	Partner, and supporter
Focus of support	Cure illness or correct incapableness	Create supportive environment and programmes
Principle	Instructive and training-focused	Interactive and supplemental support

Under these circumstances, it is important for the staff to wait for a person to make their own decision to choose a lifestyle. Staff have to respect that decision, and finds ways of offering support, so that wishes can be realised. In this sense, the staff work with users as partners.

5. A person with psychiatric disabilities is not alone. They live within the network of persons with psychiatric disabilities, and thus feel supported.
6. The life goal is to find ways in which to participate as a creative member of society through comradeship with those who share similar experiences of mental illness, or who could share similar values, rather than placing a strong stress on productivity. Through such encounters, one may find something worthwhile and significant to do in life.

Future development of Yadokarinosato

Yadokarinosato has so far only served a small group of the population: 114 members, in the city of Omiya (population: 500,000) in Saitama Prefecture. Considering the scarce range of community support service programmes that are currently offered, Yadokarinosato has provided an integrated service for its members to make community living for people with psychiatric disabilities possible for the past 25 years in Japan. Yadokarinosato has developed a support system by providing housing with support, consumers' support networks, and crisis intervention through case-management. The task is to develop a comprehensive support service system on a larger scale in the near future. We have argued that Omiya city needs one integrated service unit per 100,000 people. There is still a paucity of resources and support services in Japan, and a strong emphasis on psychiatric hospitals, which limits the opportunities to bring about the community living of persons with psychiatric disabilities. While we expect the further development of community-based services for persons with psychiatric disabilities in Japan, in the present situation we have to depend largely on volunteers. However, through building partnerships between mental health professionals, consumers, and volunteers, we may accelerate the process of normalisation, and make the community a better place to live for persons with psychiatric disabilities.

Mental health and welfare programmes in general hospitals

Health centres are becoming more and more involved in mental health activities following the recommendation made by the Ministry of Health and Welfare in January 1996. The recommendation asked health centres to play a central administrative role in the development of mental health and welfare programmes in the community. The number and scope of the mental health programmes available at a health centre depend on its resources and on the interests of staff members. A large number of staff members are public health nurses.

One of the most important programmes carried out at health centres is education for families of mentally ill people. A recent survey revealed that out of 852 health centres in Japan 509 centres (68.9%) organised educational programmes for family members of mentally ill people. In addition, 43 health centres plan to introduce family training programmes in 1997. In Hyogo Prefecture, out of 41 health centres, 30 health centres (76.9%) organised family training programmes in 1996. The content of these programmes vary. The most frequent form is a monthly lecture to family members about the nature and treatment of mental disorders. 30% used the *Handbook for families of schizophrenia* developed by the Japanese Association of Families of Mental Patients. Social skills training was carried out at about 10% of centres. A more intensive psycho-education approach was carried out at 5% of centres. Almost 20% of centres had a structured programme for family education.

Geriatric mental health and welfare services

Due to the sharp increase in the geriatric population, and changes in family structure, services for geriatric patients, particularly for senile dementia, have become the priority all over Japan.

Hyogo Prefecture has developed the following activities:

1. Consultation on geriatric mental health: consultation activities with families with senile dementia at public health centres.
2. Financial support to geriatric care centres.
3. Training for general physicians and public health nurses in the management of senile dementia.
4. Support to the in-patients rehabilitation facilities for senile dementia patients.
5. Development of comprehensive community care systems for senile dementia; including health, medical treatment and social rehabilitation.

Psychological care for the victims of the Hanshin Awaji earthquake

Local industries were severely damaged by the Hanshin Awaji earthquake, and many people who survived lost their jobs. Local government quickly built temporary houses for 80,000 people. They gradually moved to public housing and houses built with the aid of low-interest loans. At present, almost 20,000 people still live in temporary houses.

The impact of the earthquake was serious among the disadvantaged population, such as the elderly, who lost family, and who have no financial resources with which to re-build their houses. Soon after the earthquake, Hyogo Prefecture set up a Psychological Care Centre for the care of victims of the earthquake with post-traumatic stress disorder. The centre has its own building, and recruited around 30 staff members consisting of psychiatrists, psychologists and social workers. The centre provides consultation services at public health centres for victims with psychosocial problems, and services by mobile teams at temporary shelters and residences of victims.

Alcohol-related problems became serious among victims living in temporary housing. A special programme was set up for the prevention and rehabilitation of alcohol-related problems among victims. In 1996, the centre received 9516 consultations, including telephone counselling. The centre organised 97 lectures and meetings for health workers and victims to deal with PTSD and other psychological problems following the earthquake. Complaints of new cases of victims (3851) included insomnia, anxiety, PTSD symptoms, depressive feelings, mood disorders, alcohol problems, hallucinations and delusions, behavioural problems, difficulties in interpersonal relationships, and somatic symptoms. The Psychological Centre for the victims of disaster is unique to Kobe, and is expected to function for five years.

Residential facilities in the community

Rehabilitation facilities for psychiatric patients are poorly developed. The lack of rehabilitation facilities is cited as being the major factor contributing to the very long average length of stay for in-patients in Japan. Therefore, it was recommended to develop a number of rehabilitation programmes to facilitate the discharge of long-stay psychiatric patients, many of whom stay in hospital because they have no alternative place. Based on the policy of shifting the emphasis onto community care, the Ministry of Health made it a priority to increase the number of rehabilitation facilities in the community. In line with government policy, several activities to promote community programmes have been initiated in recent years in the Kobe area. They are as follows:

1. Day care activities at Prefectural mental health centres.
2. Social rehabilitation activities. Support to three life skill training homes for discharged patients unable to lead an independent life.

Each life skill training home has a capacity of 50 inmates, but actually accommodates 20–30 patients. There are only three life skill training homes in Hyogo Prefecture out of 99 in Japan at present.

3. Support to small scale occupational workshops run by the Parent Association. There are 31 small scale workshops in Hyogo. The capacity of each workshop is around 10. At national level, the government plans to increase its number from the present 563 to 686 by the year 2002.
4. Support to group homes. Group homes are for discharged patients who are able to lead independent lives in the community. There are five in Hyogo. Each group home has 5–6 patients. At the national level, it is planned to set up 3 group homes of 5–6 patients for each health and welfare unit (300,900 to 400,000 population). In Japan 920 group homes for 5060 patients will be completed by the year 2002.
5. Identification of and support for employers who provide jobs for discharged patients (occupational parents). For the rehabilitation and social integration of discharged patients, it is necessary to find industries who employ patients.
6. The rehabilitation programme for discharged patients at a welfare home. There are four welfare homes for discharged patients in Hyogo Prefecture who are able to lead independent lives but unable to find homes after their discharge from hospital. Their capacity is around 10.
7. Support to Parents Association and Alcoholics Anonymous.
8. Support to psychosocial rehabilitation activities for in-patients. National insurance schemes pay less to long-stay patients, but instead cover payment to rehabilitation programmes at hospitals.
9. Issuing of mental health and welfare card to patients. The holder of the card can get several benefits, including the use of public transportation and other public services for free or for a reduced fee.
10. Training of personnel in psychosocial rehabilitation.

Although there is increasing interest in setting up a variety of residential and non-residential rehabilitation programmes in the community, their number is very small when compared to the huge number of psychiatric beds in the hospitals. The majority of community rehabilitation programmes are established privately with a subsidy from central and local government. In the majority of cases, the running costs of community programmes are financially supported by the prefectural mental health programme.

CREATING A FOCUS UPON USERS, CARERS AND HUMAN RIGHTS

Users' organisations

Due to the strong stigma attached to mental illness, the involvement of users in the planning and evaluating of mental health services is still in a very early stage. In 1992, the National Federation of Persons with Psychiatric disabilities was established. In Japan, consumer involvement in medicine in general is very poorly developed. Informed consent for medical treatment has become an important social issue in recent years. This is especially true of the mental disorders. The weakness of consumer involvement is based on the paternalistic cultural background. In Japan, 'good mental patients' are viewed as patients who obediently follow the instructions of doctors and nurses.

In the field of medicine, equal partnership between service providers and service receivers is a long way from being achieved. Compared to the involvement of consumers, the Patients Family Association (Zenkaren) has been active and vocal. Zenkaren has contributed to the improvement of psychiatric care in Japan. Besides the user's organisation of people with mental illness, there are a few other consumer activities worth mentioning.

First is the movement of Alcoholics Anonymous (AA) Japan which has a relatively long history. At present almost all prefectures have AA.

Second is the self-help group of Morita Neurotic Patients. Morita neurosis is considered to be a kind of social phobia specific to Asian culture. The group is called Seikatu-no-Hakken-Kai (Life Discovering Association). They have around 6000 members and issue their own journals. They meet once a month to study principles of living skills, and to exchange their experiences of adapting to their daily life. Morita therapy was developed by Professor M Morita, a Japanese psychiatrist, about 80 years ago, based on his experience of curing his own neurosis. Morita therapy is said to be based on the living principles of Zen and Taoism.

Support to consumer and family involvement

In Japan, the Association of Families with Mental Patients runs occupational training centres for patients. Also, they have published a booklet for the education of family members on mental illness which is now used at health centres. Consumer involvement is very low key in Japan, even for ordinary illnesses. Asia has a rather authoritative culture where the medical profession has an unquestionable right over the patient. Only recently has informed consent for cancer treatment become a social issue in Japan. Consumer involvement in mental health will be an important area to be promoted in Japan and in the city of Kobe in the future.

Protection of human rights of people with mental illness

The Mental Hygiene Law was revised in Japan in 1988 and renamed as the Mental Health Law. Mental health law in Japan has a focus on the protection of human rights of people with mental illnesses and the promotion of community-based services for them. The spirit of these laws is the same as similar laws in USA and Europe. However, there are a few differences reflecting culture and value. In Japan, hospitalisation by consent of the family members has been legally approved even after the revision of Mental Health law in 1988. Hospitalisation based on consent by a family member (mostly father or mother) has been renamed as hospitalisation based on medical protection. The value and authority attached to families in Asian countries are not the same as in Europe and USA. The communal orientation is far stronger than individual value in traditional Asian societies. The legal basis for compulsory treatment in Japan could be different from that in USA and Europe. However, it will be important for Japanese mental health professionals to follow due legal process to protect the human rights of people with mental illness in Japan.

SERVICE EVALUATION

Each prefecture has its own local mental health commission. Hyogo Prefecture Government has Hyogo Prefectural Mental Health Commission as an advisory body. Members include psychiatrists, professors, welfare officers, representatives of the Family Association and representatives of the Employers Association of discharged patients. The commission has a mandate to protect the human rights of people with mental illness. It reviews requests for compulsory admission and medical protection admission. Also, the commission reviews requests for the discharge of patients, as well as the human rights of in-patients.

In 1989, the Ministry of Health and Welfare and the Japanese Medical Association developed a 'Hospital Function Evaluation Manual' with a view to improving the quality of hospital services. This was adopted by the Japanese Private Psychiatric Hospital Association (Nisseikyo), and Nisseikyo prepared the 'Psychiatric Hospital Function Evaluation Manual' in 1990. In 1993, a peer review was initiated by Nisseikyo. The review items included such items as 'quality of service', 'nursing care' and 'patient satisfaction and security'. So far, service evaluation is limited to in-patient services. The author is not aware of an evaluation scheme which will cover community care. This will be an area for further development in Japan, as well as in the Kobe area.

FUTURE DEVELOPMENTS

Demographic changes and future need

It is noteworthy that the average life span is the longest in Japan, 80 on average (76 male; 82 female). In addition, it is expected that this number will continue to increase and one-fifth of the Japanese population will be more than 60 years within 20 years. This clearly shows the importance of geriatric mental health in coming years in Japan as well as for the city of Kobe.

Decrease of in-patient psychiatric beds by developing community services

At present, Japan has the largest number of psychiatric beds in both absolute and relative number per population. In 1996, the number of psychiatric in-patients was 340,785, by far the biggest in number in the world. The lack of a community support system and stigma attached to people with mental illness promoted the hospital-based care for them. These are cited as major causes of a very long-stay for in-patients and the violation of human rights at mental hospitals in Japan. In 1997, more than half of the in-patients had stayed at psychiatric hospitals for more than five years. More than 100,000 patients, one-third of the in-patients, stay more than 10 years at psychiatric hospitals. Therefore, the priority for the future will be to reduce these long-stays for patients. This could be achieved by the introduction of various community programmes.

However, the change of the national insurance scheme would be the most important. This policy change will require a careful negotiation with the Private Psychiatric Hospital Association. At present, Japan has 27.3 psychiatric beds per 10,000 population. This figure should be reduced gradually, to be replaced by community services. In the past 10 to 20 years, many developed countries have reduced the in-patient beds to between a half and a quarter of present levels. These figures will certainly give possible answers to the number of psychiatric beds needed in Japan and in the city of Kobe. A number of 4 to 5 psychiatric beds per 10,000 population seem adequate in countries when sufficient community services are provided.

Quality control of private psychiatric hospitals

In Japan the majority of psychiatric beds are owned by the private sector. However, the clients of these hospitals are almost the same as those at hospitals owned by the government, and payments for patients at private hospitals are covered by public expenditures or national insurance schemes. In this sense, private hospitals in Japan could be classified as privately managed public services. Psychiatric services in Japan received international criticisms because of several cases of violation of human rights at private psychiatric hospitals. This has resulted in a revision of the Mental Health Law in 1988 which now focuses on community services and more attention to human rights of in-patients. Quality control of private psychiatric hospitals is the important initiative to be introduced in Japan and in the city of Kobe.

Change of financing scheme in mental health services

Out of 11,472 patients hospitalised in psychiatric hospitals in Hyogo Prefecture, fees for more than half of the in-patients are covered by national insurance schemes. The rest were covered by various schemes of public expenditures. One of the characteristics of the financing system in Japan is the point system. Any kind of treatment and care has its own financial points. Government can influence the *modus operandi* of mental health services through the manipulation of the point system. In the past, the point system sometimes gave incentives for business minded psychiatric hospitals to keep as many patients as long as possible.

In order to promote community-based programmes, the government has introduced financing measures to favour community-based programmes, such as higher payment to day care services and to home visits by nurses. Also, several innovative measures have been introduced to discourage a long stay. If a patient stays longer, the payment for in-patient care decreases. This gives an incentive for psychiatric hospitals to avoid a long stay of patients. Who and how to pay for mental health services will shape the future of mental health services in Japan and in Kobe. Therefore, it is important to introduce a financing system favouring community care.

Support for the development of private psychiatric clinics

An important recent trend in Japan is the rapid increase of private psychiatric clinics (in principle, no beds). This has been promoted due to the following reasons:

1. The stigma attached to mental illness has decreased and the public in general have less hesitation in consulting psychiatric clinics. This decrease of stigma has guaranteed sufficient numbers of out-patients to psychiatric clinics.

2. Government approved a financial incentive to psychiatric clinics increasing the payment to consultation and day care services. Also, young psychiatrists prefer to set up their own clinics rather than be employed at a private psychiatric hospital.

At present, there are 2644 private psychiatric clinics in Japan and 92 at Hyogo Prefecture which has a population of 5.5 million. On average, each private clinic has 50-70 patients a day. In addition, the number of private clinics is increasing very rapidly and private clinics will become a major vehicle to provide mental health services in the community. At the same time, the increase of private clinics would surely contribute to the further reduction of the stigma attached to mental illness.

The stigma to mental illnesses will decrease when they are treated like other chronic diseases at out-patient clinics. The best way to reduce stigma to mental illnesses will be to increase their treatment in the community. This could be realised through the introduction of a financing system favouring community care. Therefore, it will be beneficial to support the establishments of private clinics in Japan and in the city of Kobe.

Promoting mental health activities as part of public health services

In Japan, health centres are more and more involved in mental health activities after the recommendation was made by the Ministry of Health in January 1996. The recommendation asked health centres in Japan (852 in total) to play a central administrative role to develop mental health programmes in the community. Average health centres serve a population around 100,000 to 150,000. One of the important programmes carried out at general health centres has been education for families of the mentally ill. These developments at health centres should be promoted as a positive step to promote community-based mental health services in Japan.

CHAPTER EIGHT

The city of Madison, USA The Madison Model: keeping the focus of treatment in the community

David LeCount
Dane County Department of Mental Health, Madison, USA

THE CITY OF MADISON, USA

The July 1996 issue of *Money Magazine* ranked Madison, Wisconsin, as the best place to live in America based on its vibrant economy (1.7% unemployment rate and plentiful jobs), excellent health care and educational systems, and low crime rate (Fried, 1996). In addition to being a great place to live and work, it is also a community that has a rich tradition of working together in solving problems. Madison achieved the highest ranking in health care which is largely provided through four primary managed care companies called Health Maintenance Organisations. Located in south-central Wisconsin, Madison is home of the state capitol, and makes up approximately half of the 390,000 residents of Dane County. Surrounded by plentiful lakes, dairy farms and biking trails, the half-mile-wide isthmus with the Capitol at the centre is where the core public mental health programmes exist in proximity to most of the consumers of mental health services. It is against this backdrop that the adult mental health system has evolved over the past 23 years.

THE ADULT MENTAL HEALTH SYSTEM

The Madison Model

An advantage of living in Madison has been the leadership role played by excellent community oriented psychiatrists in generalising research into practical application within the context of community-based treatment. In the community of Madison the concept of the 'dignity of risk' has taken on great significance in the total evolution of the system. Psychiatrists have assumed the primary leadership in the development and sanctioning of the Dane County (Madison) system. The senior psychiatrists have taught the psychiatric residents concepts of community psychiatry and inter-disciplinary teamwork to maximise community integration. The Mental Health Centre of Dane County (MHCDC) has provided *in vivo* training in their core psychiatric programmes for these residents. Many of these psychiatrists have continued to work in this model following their training, as well as carrying on the tradition in other parts of the country and world. We credit the contributions of community oriented psychiatrists with significant research findings and practical applications as well as pioneering approaches reflected throughout this report. Indeed, many of the primary philosophical principles that are a hallmark of this system have been developed and promoted by these seminal psychiatrists.

Programme of assertive community treatment (PACT)

Since 1974, the adult mental health system administered by Dane County has received widespread recognition and replication, and has evolved to its current form: a comprehensive and integrated continuum of managed care for persons who have a serious and persistent mental illness. The Program of Assertive Community Treatment (PACT), begun in 1972, was a precursor to the core continuous treatment teams currently administered through the county's system of care. The PACT programme demonstrated the efficacy of community-based treatment by 1978, and many of its proven treatment strategies have been generalised to the larger system in its present form. Since 1980, most of the community support programmes (CSPs) are now provided through the mental health centre of Dane County's four programmes serving 350 clients. As a state administered out-patient programme, PACT continues to be a part of the Madison Model, representing one of the 40 programmes currently under contract with the Dane County Department of Human Services. It provides services to 133 of the 1537 clients who qualify as having the most serious and persistent mental illnesses. Additionally, many single element programmes continue to operate, but all are held together through contracted relationships, central entry points, and fixed case management responsibilities. Today the entire system of care is referenced as an integrated community support system.

The PACT programme, as a pioneer and prototype model, is well known for demonstrating that in utilising a continuous treatment team, most clients can be stabilised and treated in the community, hence minimising the need for periodic and repeated hospitalisations. This program's control group, which receives primary treatment from the Dane County system, currently more closely approximates the results of the PACT programme, particularly in regard to decreased levels of psychiatric hospitalisations.

PACT pioneered comprehensive and continuous community-based treatment referred to as Training in Community Living (TCL) of Continuous Treatment Team (CTT), for persons with serious and persistent mental illness. Diagnostically, these include schizophrenia, schizoaffective, major affective disorders, or severe personality disorders. Their research in using this model and comparing it to a control group focused initially (1972–1978) on people who were 18–62 years old. From 1978 to the present time, the age range has been 18–30 for persons with dual disabilities, substance abuse, and serious and persistent mental illness. The control group has been primarily other Dane County public mental health system contracted services, which have become more refined over time.

Research findings are similar for all ages treated. Comprehensive, continuous assertive community-based treatment through TCL compared with the control group resulted in the TCL participants experiencing less use of hospitalisation, spending more time in independent living, manifesting fewer symptoms, having more involvement in employment, and experiencing a greater satisfaction with life (Stein, Test, & Marx 1975; Stein & Test, 1978, 1980; Test & Stein, 1978; Industry Profile, 1988). In an earlier economic cost-benefit analysis study, it was concluded that the cost for hospital-based and community-based treatment were the same: $7200 per patient per year (Weisbrod, Test, & Stein, 1980).

In addition to the PACT research findings, the entire Dane County adult mental health system is now viewed as a national model of good community care (Stein, Diamond & Factor 1992). For many years the PACT programme has had a 'work as treatment' emphasis which is considered to be a crucial part of the psychiatric rehabilitation process. There are now seven vocational specialists in the PACT programme and they have been able to maintain over 50% of their clients in competitive jobs (Frey, 1994). The next phase in the PACT research is to work with an even younger age range, 15–21. This is a logical progression in keeping with past emphasis on moving towards the earliest onset of the illness. They have concluded that some of the clients in their current group (ages 18–30) may have been identified earlier, and with comprehensive treatment may not have lost functional impairment due to being out of school, and by having better management of symptoms and reduction of episodic in-patient treatment.

A national community support training resource centre

The National Institute of Mental Health (NIMH) has designated Dane County's system of care a 'National community support training resource centre'. Mental health professionals throughout the world have received training from the many programmes in Madison. Thompson, Griffith, and Philip (1990) concluded 'the success of the experimental clinical trials and imprimatur of NIMH have led many programme planners to see the Madison Model of community care as a basic structure on which to build their own public mental health care systems. In addition, the experience of Dane County frequently serves as a reference point for measuring the achievements of other systems of care'. Torrey and Wolfe (1986) stated: 'Wisconsin has achieved a national reputation for excellent services for the seriously mentally ill primarily on the basis of the programmes in a single county—Dane County'.

Ironically, even though the PACT prototype and the Madison Model have been widely studied, evaluated, and disseminated, there are many aspects of their programmatic success that remain unique and are not well publicised or understood. Since its inception 23 years ago, the Madison Model has maintained a focus on community treatment. The following highlights reflect how this emphasis has been maintained.

A centralised agency with fixed responsibility for total management and oversight

One of the most distinguishing features in the Dane County system is that the primary oversight of the entire public system is fixed in one central agency, which significantly enhances the ability to provide a well coordinated system of care. The Wisconsin State Statute dealing with disabilities, 'Chapter 51', was revised in the early 1970s to reflect the change from hospital to community as the focal point of treatment. This comprehensive legislation mandated that counties be responsible for the planning, development, budgeting, delivery, monitoring, and evaluation of mental health services relegated to the public sector. Chapter 51 included a patients' Bill of Rights section, specifying that treatment should occur in the least restrictive environment, providing for a dangerousness standard and due process for involuntary treatment.

All court ordered services then became a mandated responsibility for the counties to implement and it required counties to pay for all services including in-patient treatment. Chapter 51 changed the status of state hospitals, and further specified that all services be authorised and statistically reported, tracked, and evaluated.

Target population. Within a period between 1974 and 1980, it became clear that the public sector's primary responsibility was to those most in need who required a system of care not previously available. The Alliance for the Mentally Ill of Dane County (AMI) provided an additional impetus to clarify who should receive services. Today, over 1500 persons with the most severe schizophrenic and affective disorders receive the preponderance of the services, and another approximately 3000 people receive more limited interventions. Many other people with dual mental health and substance abuse disorders and multiple disabilities are also the public sector's responsibility.

System management. Dane County has always elected to contract for services based on the cost savings this represents and the availability of well qualified existing private, non-profit agencies such as the Mental Health Centre of Dane County. Today there are 17 different agencies and 40 programmes providing services through this contractual arrangement creating a public-private partnership.

Cost and clinical effectiveness

The Madison Model has from its inception had to cope with limited funding and risk liability by developing a system of care that is both cost effective and clinically effective. A conscious-guiding principle has been to emphasise concurrently therapeutic interventions that are effective, requiring the system to work in tandem with all related networks to maximise its efficiencies.

Every aspect of the system has been created and designed with the concept of cost effectiveness and clinical soundness in mind. As stated in an article reviewing the history of the Madison Model: 'The ultimate stated goal of the system is to provide the least expensive mix of services necessary to enable each patient to live in the community, minimising patients' relapses while maximising their independence and quality of life'. (Thompson et al. 1990).

Most services were planned and developed with the assumption that community-based alternatives would reduce the need for high-cost in-patient services. In reality, it took until 1981 before this dream was realised. At that point, monies saved were realigned into community services. However, even with maintaining the average length of stay at 15 days over the past 10 years, the cost of in-patient care at the state hospital has increased dramatically from a rate of $78 per day in 1978 versus $551 today. The present annual cost of care for one patient at the Mendota Mental Health Institute (the state hospital located in Madison) comes to $201,115. With a current budget of $13,244,100 to serve 1537 people who have serious and persistent mental illnesses, the average cost per person is approximately $7324. Over a year's time, 27 people can be served in the community for the same cost as one person on an in-patient basis. While over 4000 people receive some level of service in the adult mental health system, approximately 85% of the funding goes for services to people most in need and most severely impaired.

Contracting for services was a conscious decision made early on because of the numerous and well qualified private non-profit human service agencies already available in the Madison community. Studies indicated that in many instances the county can provide services at a reduced cost by outsourcing. The contracted system provides a wide range of cost-effective services throughout this stratified continuum in the following ways. All of these factors provide services to more people at lower cost, fostering both effective treatment in the community as well as ongoing recovery.

Minimising costs. The high cost institutional centres have been minimised. Core psychiatric services are provided through the Mental Health Centre of Dane County, and many other case management, work services, and programmes that emphasised psychosocial and functional needs are being provided at a lower cost by other providers.

Community care. As stated above, most of the community-based programmes have been added over the years to reduce hospital utilisation, not only from a cost and treatment standpoint, but also because of client preference and to meet court-ordered requirements mandating the least restrictive treatment environment. The development of the community support programmes and supervised living arrangements has significantly contributed towards this end. For example, for one programme alone, Crisis Homes, the coordinator estimated that 483 in-patient days had been avoided during 1996, achieving a net cost savings of $258,567 for the system.

Drug services. Due to the decline in number of private practitioners serving persons on Medical Assistance (a federal/state insurance programme), cost-effective solutions were developed to provide more psychotropic drug services for persons unable to access the private sector. Over 400 additional persons gained access to psychotropic drugs with the creation of a separate medications unit, called the Medical Services Unit, at the mental health centre, where nurses with R.N. degrees and psychiatrists efficiently serve individuals requiring psychotropics. More recently an increase in the number of people receiving psychotropics has been achieved with psychiatrists consulting at family practice clinics (primary health care centres staffed by general practitioners serving

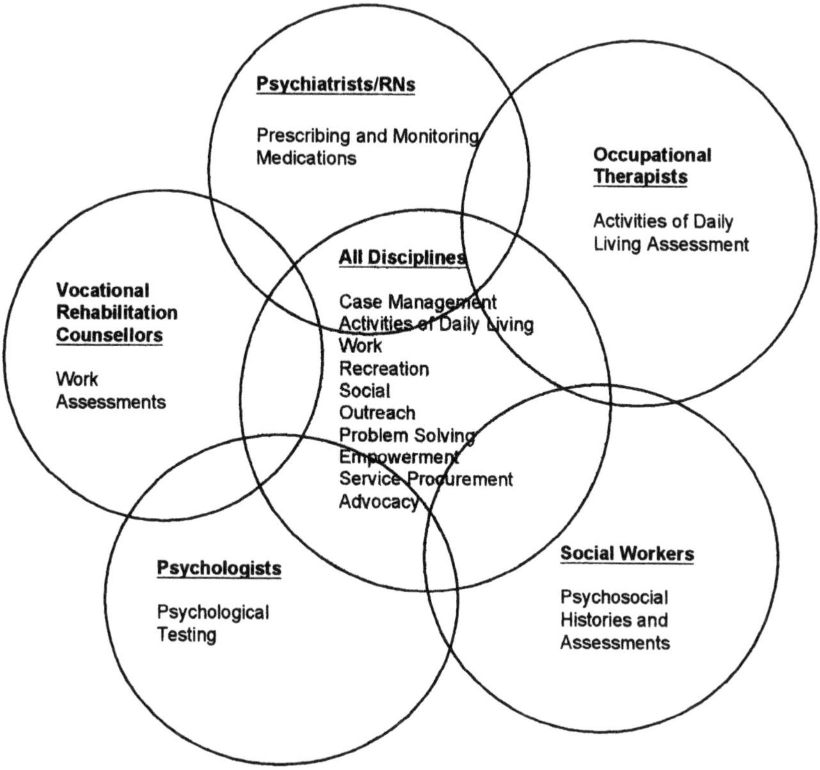

FIG. 8.1. Role delineation/role blurring.

low-income persons) and psychiatric residents providing a medications clinic at a homeless shelter.

Role delineation and blurring. Role delineation is well defined in the system so cost effectiveness can be achieved with greater treatment efficiencies. Correspondingly, the concept of role blurring (generalists) has been incorporated into the subculture of the human services delivery system and related networks (Fig. 8.1). While case management functions and psychosocial interventions within mental health cross many disciplines, there is a great amount of respect for the particular expertise that each profession brings to the treatment process. It is understood that specialised functions such as making diagnoses, performing psychological testing, prescribing psychotropic medications, ruling out nonpsychiatric medical issues, performing mental status exams, and assessing work/living/general functioning all require specialised training, expertise, licensure, and certification. Whereas, helping clients learn new coping mechanisms and problem solving skills is not only relegated to the psychotherapist, but is a part of the everyday communication process with clients across all disciplines. Role delineation occurs in many ways. The work time of psychiatric personnel is always at a premium, and so it is used primarily in a medically necessary and cost-effective manner. Psychiatric physicians, along with psychiatric nurses, focus on the psychotropic drug needs of clients. Psychiatrists complete psychiatric workups and make referrals to other medical specialities as needed. In addition to being consultants to treatment teams, psychiatrists also endorse and respect the roles of all other involved professionals. In the Emergency Services Unit, psychiatric social workers, nurses, and other personnel complete crisis assessments and involve a psychiatrist only as needed. Vocational rehabilitation counsellors may initiate work assessment and placement with ongoing support being provided by the employer or another staff member. In some programmes, occupational therapists take the lead in assessing Activities of Daily Living (ADLs) skills. However, all staff can assist in teaching skills for living successfully in the community. Table 8.1 shows the number of staff by discipline per 100,000 population.

Self-help peer support. Client (peer) support is being incorporated into the various facets of our treatment network on a paid and volunteer basis. Clients are employed in supervised living settings, the Emergency Services Unit, and community support programmes. A minimum of seven client operated organisations also function independently from the existing contracted system. Other self-help peer support groups are incorporated into existing programmes such as Yahara House. The AMI has numerous ongoing support groups for consumers and affected family members, and also provide educational programmes such as 'Journey of Hope'. Consumers are involved in planning and hiring processes and serve on provider boards and other decision making committees. Natural support systems are encouraged and supported throughout the system.

TABLE 8.1
Number of Staff by Discipline per 100,000 Population

Staff by Discipline	*Total*	*Per 100,000*
Psychiatrists	10	2.50
Registered nurses	45	11.25
Social work and/or related Master's degree staff	70	17.50
Licensed psychologists	3	0.75
Bachelor's degree staff	80	20.00
Non-degree clinical staff (Mental health technicians)	30	7.50
Total	228	59.50

A mature system of care

Deinstitutionalisation has been largely accomplished after many years, with over 95% of the clients now living in the community and receiving some degree of community-based services. Most of the county mental health clients reside in integrated scattered site apartments while receiving external support. As a result, they have become more fully integrated into the community. Contrasted with their predecessors, the current generation of mental health clients have not experienced the great degree of institutionalisation and its related problems such as dependency and missed opportunities.

Maturity of care has also occurred through the budget expenditures and distribution as it provides a comprehensive continuum of care exemplified in Table 8.2. For many years, over 80% of the funding has gone for community-based treatment, with less than 20% for in-patient psychiatric treatment. This is with the belief that the community is the most therapeutic environment, providing the greatest potential for self-fulfilment. In its present form this funding distribution represents a balanced and stable system of care that is to be maintained. If cost overruns are seen in in-patient accounts, further analyses are made to determine needed corrections, either through system change or programmatic enhancements. Presently, as the system is at capacity, the challenge is in dealing with both extensive waiting lists and increasing in-patient costs.

The maturity of the system is shown in the funding realignments that have occurred since the early days. The primary redistribution initially

TABLE 8.2
Budget Expenditures and Distribution

Expenditures	*Amount*	*Percent*
Community support programmes	3,570,600	29.96
Living arrangements	2,884,200	21.78
Case management	1,481,400	11.19
In-patient		
Acute/Involuntary State Hosp.	855,800	6.46
Acute/Voluntary Comm. Hosp.	320,200	2.42
Long-term in-patient	889,000	6.71
Crisis intervention	1,073,700	8.11
Psychotherapy	774,800	5.85
Work-related services	484,400	3.66
Day services	462,200	3.49
Outreach/Miscellaneous	393,900	3.97
Med. Serv. Unit-Medications	53,900	0.41
Total expenditures	$13,244,100	100%

occurred by decreasing the funding for psychiatric in-patient services and providing more money for community-based services. Contract performance decisions have guided other funding realignments, as well as the inability of certain programmes to meet the county's requirement of an integrated system of care. In all instances, these realignments have positively enhanced treatment programmes. A representative example of this was the start up of the Crisis Home and Short-Term Care programmes in 1988 by diverting funds from a high cost group home that had become more of a permanent than a transitional setting.

If clients cannot receive more intensive services on a proactive basis in the community because the system is at capacity, they will probably require hospitalisation. Further, if the highly structured supervised living arrangement system is not mobile, or if too many clients are hospitalised at any given time, they may have to wait longer in an in-patient psychiatric facility for community-based alternatives to be arranged. To date the system has been able to maintain this delicate balance despite remaining somewhat precarious.

An integrated and multi-tiered system of care

The system has evolved since the original description by Mosher & Burti (1989) to a three level system to define more clearly how services are matched with needs. This is very much in keeping with principles of managed care.

Level I: Integrated, comprehensive core services. These programmes are the most staff intensive, providing assertive outreach and continuous treatment approaches by dealing with clients at the highest risk for hospitalisation. The clinicians working at this level become keenly aware of 'soft' signs of deterioration, and therefore are more assertive in their treatment stabilisation efforts. This level requires all or most services to be consolidated within a single treatment team. In addition to the PACT programme, there are five CSP teams provided through four programmes at the Mental Health Centre of Dane County. Day services are modelled after the 'Fountain House' programme with psychosocial and vocational emphases. The psychiatric in-patient continuum includes Badger Prairie Health Care Centre (a county nursing home for long-term in-patient treatment), Mendota Mental Health Institute (a state-operated involuntary acute treatment centre), and three community hospitals with psychiatric wards (for voluntary acute treatment). System case management is provided for 650 people at this level.

Level II: Multiple single service programmes. This level of programming is available for clients who are less vulnerable to relapse and able to engage with multiple service providers to have their needs met. They may have a case manager through one programme, receive medications through another, and participate in an altogether separate work programme. Twenty-four hour response is available through the Emergency Services Unit. Psychotropic medications are provided by the Medical Services Unit. Four agencies offer short-term solution focused psychotherapy. All 40 programmes provide case management services, but a Community Intervention Team performs this function exclusively at this level. While supported employment services are available through the CSPs and day service programme, three other programmes provide only work-related services. The internal supervised living arrangement system consists of 201 supervised living arrangements with 102 group home slots in multiple sites, nine crisis home slots, seven short-term care slots, 35 adult family home settings, and some individualised living arrangements. Thirty-eight slots are provided in three congregate apartments and three boarding homes, all of which offer minimal staff support. While most of the programmes at this level provide only a primary service, there are some exceptions. One example is the Mobile Outreach to Seniors Team (MOST), which offers case management, psychotherapy/psychotropics, and consultation services to the county's coalitions for the aging. System case management is provided for 673 people at this level.

Level III: Services that integrate homeless and 'unconnected' people. Here the goals are to first meet basic needs (food, clothing, and shelter) and then prepare clients for treatment. In some instances they may require involuntary treatment services. The main function of this level is outreach. Programmes here meet basic needs (food, clothing, and shelter) and attempt to connect people with mental health services through either a relationship approach or an involuntary process. Some of the programmes/services here include homeless shelters, a transitional housing programme, outreach workers, a medications clinic, and representative payees. Since the core treatment programmes were established in 1986, the County has been concentrating more of its contracts with the basic needs network and has established monthly system coordination meetings to focus on getting more of these people into treatment. Staff working at this level are not referred to as 'case managers', but are considered the *primary contact workers* even though they perform similar functions such as procuring services and building relationships. Primary contact workers serve 214 persons. Other related networks and agencies are involved, such as law enforcement, emergency response systems, and the Social Security Administration.

Service according to needs. Clients are served at all levels and can rotate among these three tiers depending upon needs and their ability to be maintained within this system of care. Treatment expectations vary based upon the degree of staff intensity available in each programme, which is dependent upon the size of case loads and amount of time that can be devoted to each client. This levels system allows flexibility and change to occur in a more orderly fashion. While the goal of the system is to maintain high need clients within the most appropriate level of care, it is recognised that clients are highly mobile and the system must respond to both positive and negative changes in their condition.

Major service areas in the system

Community support programmes. Service progression: from PACT demonstrated research to system integration. Although the entire system is viewed as a community support programme with many variations on this theme, for the purposes of this section, CSPs will be discussed in relation to the continuous, interdisciplinary treatment teams. Here the majority of their comprehensive services are delivered in the community rather than in programme offices.

Since the inception of the county system with the PACT approach arising as the most effective model for persons at highest risk of repeated in-patient treatment, the key variables have been timing, prioritisation, funding, and means of implementation. The state worked in conjunction with the Alliance for the Mentally Ill to realise PACT's implementation on a system-wide basis. The first steps were obtaining a CSP funding initiative in 1980 and obtaining Medical Assistance funding. Almost one-third of the clients (approximately 483 people) receive services through five programmes representing six continuous treatment teams.

There are many features of the community support programme. An interdisciplinary team provides assertive and comprehensive services, mostly in the community (*in vivo*) to address the psychiatric and functional impairments of those most seriously mentally ill. The team treats mental illness symptoms with somatic and behavioural therapy and teaches clients awareness and self-management of those symptoms. They provide behavioural, supportive, and teaching strategies for dealing with functional deficits, such as limitations in social, vocational, and coping skills, and activities of daily living (ADLs) to enhance successful living in the community. The staff intensity of the CSP allows an increase in service delivery during periods of higher illness acuity. Staff-to-client ratios range from 1:8 to 1:13. Outcomes focus on low hospitalisation rates (25% or less), symptom stabilisation, independent living, and paid employment. In addition, one

CSP, Community Treatment Alternatives, which only accepts clients directly from the Dane County jail, has reduced jail recidivism by nearly 70%.

Community support programmes have proven their worth, viability, and cost effectiveness. More CSP slots are needed. Many people continually enter the system and cannot access CSP services, while others are underserved in existing single service programmes. Even though PACT has demonstrated the effectiveness of the assertive community treatment approach since 1978, 70% of public funding in the broader United States continues to fund in-patient treatment. The National Alliance for the Mentally Ill is currently working to institute the PACT model and its standards throughout the nation.

Living arrangements. Service progression: from substandard apartments and inexpensive hotels to supported-living arrangements to integrated apartments. Dane County has progressed significantly from the days of discharging people from hospital settings directly to large, congregate hotels and other semi-supervised residences, to now providing supportive living environments in the community. The closing of a large residential care centre in 1982 with 166 beds was an opportunity to create more individualised and consumer-friendly living environments; three additional group homes, an adult foster home programme, and other less intensive supervised living arrangements were developed through special funding. The goal was to optimise community integration by individualising and supervising community living.

Today approximately 88% of clients live in their own apartments with external staff support. Twelve percent live in a facility having internal staff supervision operated by or contracted with the county. The latter includes 35 persons in a county nursing home, 102 in group homes, and 48 in adult family homes and other individualised settings (Table 8.3). Almost all of these 185 users will progress to their own apartments eventually. The

TABLE 8.3
Supervised Housing (1996 Data)

High to Low Structure	*Slots*	*Served*
9 Group homes	82	93
1 Receiving centre	20	139
9 Crisis homes	9	182
3 Short-term care homes	3	40
35 Adult family homes	35	48
3 Boarding homes	12	16
4 Congregate apartments	40	45
Totals	201	563

evolution of client housing from an array of supervised transitional living to a well stratified system of higher to lower structure is shown in the following chart. There are at present no set time periods for clients to remain in staff supported settings. Currently group homes with the highest level of staff support are used primarily by clients coming out of in-patient settings. The supervised living arrangements are mainly transitional and are used as a means toward the end goal of clients living independently with external support.

With the development of a continuum of treatment services, providers and clients have promoted quality, scattered-site housing instead of the large congregate buildings constructed by the public housing authorities. Federal Housing and Urban Development (HUD) and county funding, combined with existing staff support (case management services), have allowed supervised and quality independent apartments to be provided since that time. The timing of our improvements coincided with the change in HUD emphasis from solely constructing living quarters to the inclusion of services to assist in more successful independent living. A private non-profit agency, Housing Initiatives, was incorporated to disseminate rent subsidies (whereby the client pays 30% of his/her income for rent), enabling 70 persons to reside in higher quality apartments integrated throughout the community.

A recent development is the incorporation into the system of a 'Housing Resource Specialist' within the central entry point to track the availability of affordable housing that best meets client preferences. Both clients and providers are kept informed of the available housing stock. In this manner, community integration will further evolve, with the ultimate goal being home ownership.

Case management. Service progression: from a single designation within a programme to system-wide designation across multiple programmes. Case management is the glue that holds the system together. In its purest form, case management functions encompass everything from assessment, treatment of symptoms, rehabilitation planning, interventions, and ongoing evaluation, to coordination and advocacy services for linkage and referrals. As staff-to-client ratios increase, the expectations become less pronounced. Levels I and II adhere to the purest form of case management. However, in Level III, the primary contact staff provide outreach services to meet basic needs and work over time to connect clients with treatment. Case managers do not necessarily provide all the services, but must see that all aspects of the treatment/rehabilitation programmes are implemented within their programme and across all other involved programmes.

Emergency services. Service progression: from crisis intervention to system-wide functions emphasising community-based treatment. The nerve centre of the adult mental health system is the Emergency Services Unit (ESU), which started in 1968 in response to dictates from the courts. ESU's functions have expanded since then, especially in response to system demands. This energised unit works like a beehive, exemplifying the essence of creative problem solving at all levels. Staff at ESU interact with law enforcement personnel and an endless number of other community resources. They work particularly hard to strengthen natural supports of the client, sometimes serve to fill gaps in the system, and although they can provide mobile services, generally respond to clients over the phone or as walk-ins. ESU is efficient and effective, with its focus always on the community as the primary treatment environment. Essential to maintaining its community emphasis during crisis triage dispositions is its operation as an independent unit apart from a hospital setting.

ESU was initially designated as the gatekeeper or entity for authorising in-patient hospital admissions. It was not until 1980 that its functions were broadened to include ongoing monitoring, facilitating, and implementing after-care placements for all authorised admissions. This approach has more effectively minimised the use of hospitalisation, and ensures that out-patient alternatives to admission are fully exploited. According to ESU's 1996 outcome data, 67% of the 1413 requests for hospitalisation were diverted to community treatment alternatives, many of which included follow-up of the client in the crisis unit or placement in a crisis home. True creativity emerges when ESU staff respond to a person experiencing stress and anxiety by capturing what the clients want and need to help them cope. Sometimes this means just having the client be with a friend or family member or other natural supports.

Staff at ESU have a unique relationship with the police, and this involves mutual training. A clear definition of roles exists in that the police define alleged dangerousness and ESU staff determine mental status, while both work toward an end disposition. This level of triage produces the most clinically and cost-effective disposition and conforms to the statutory requirements of least-restrictive alternatives. Policy at the Madison Police Department is that all persons potentially needing psychiatric hospitalisation, or who appear to be in a mental health crisis, be taken to the ESU for assessment and assistance in disposition.

ESU monitors civil commitments and settlement agreements to ensure that treatment requirements are met. As a part of this process, they also write a report to the court before the expiration of the commitment specifying their recommendations regarding extension or lapsing of the commitment. Crisis alerts can be established with ESU largely through the provider system when it is known a client is decompensating and may be needing a higher level response. Staff at ESU then work with the referring source to see that all voluntary out-patient alternatives are applied.

ESU provides an all important 24–hour phone service for all eligible Dane County citizens needing a mental health response or experiencing a mental health crisis. ESU also provides an on-site staff linkage to the homeless shelters thereby facilitating entry into the mental health system.

Crisis homes, which are certified adult family home sponsors, are under the direction of ESU and are frequently used instead of hospitalisation altogether or to shorten the length of in-patient stay. Of all crisis home placements, approximately 40% are in lieu of a hospital admission, 40% facilitate an earlier discharge from the hospital, and 20% represent a pre-crisis intervention or some sort of housing issue. Recent feedback from client participation in crisis homes shows a high degree of satisfaction with the home-like atmosphere of crisis homes. Clients identified two features that helped them: 'time out from a stressful situation' and 'being treated like a normal person'. Present day clients who have not experienced years of institutionalisation do not see the psychiatric hospital as the only safe and secure setting for them when their symptoms become acute. Rather, they welcome the crisis home (living temporarily with a typical family unit), along with ESU backup, as an alternative to hospitalisation.

An ESU programme used by the entire community is the 'Survivors of Suicide' (SOS) support group for the significant others affected by the suicide or sudden death of a loved one. The support of peers and ESU staff helps to enhance coping after a tragic death and personal loss.

Finally, because the system is at capacity, many times the only way a person in urgent need of psychotropic medications can be served is through ESU. In addition to backing up mental health centre programmes after hours, this is another way emergency services backs up the entire system.

In-patient continuum. Service progression: from uncontrolled in-patient usage to authorised and closely monitored in-patient tracking. Many levels of severity of illness are successfully and responsibly managed in the community. However, authorisation for in-patient hospital admission is granted when ESU staff have determined that the level of severity requires a hospital setting and the presenting disorder can be appropriately treated therein. Two standards are followed: (1) in-patient treatment is used only when it is effective for the presenting problem and (2) all other out-patient treatments have been ruled out. Usually this means in-patient placement primarily for stabilisation of acute symptoms and for titrating psychotropic medication. An in-patient exceeding the average length of stay signals a special placement problem which requires a review at all levels to ensure that either in-patient treatment is still warranted or all attempts to procure an alternative are being fully explored.

Dane County residents currently have available 97 beds per 100,000 population at risk, of which 38 are in general hospitals, 7 in the state

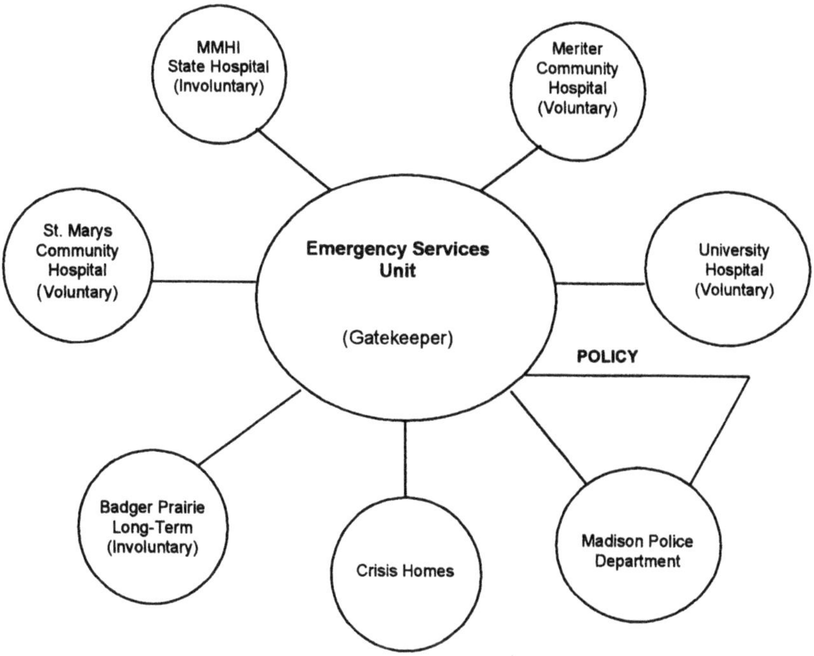

FIG. 8.2. Psychiatric in-patient continuum.

hospital, and 52 in longer term facilities. Between 1981 and 1996, the number of admissions per year to these beds has risen from 72 to 117, while the mean length of stay has dropped from 39 days to 14 days. In-patient treatments range from short-term voluntary hospitalisation in community hospitals (average stay is five days) to longer-term involuntary hospitalisations at the state hospital.

Longer term placements also occur at the Badger Prairie Health Care Centre (average stay one year). This has 35 clients in the locked ward under a court-ordered, protective placement. Approximately one-half of these will be discharged to the community during the course of a year with the goal of all eventually returning to the community. Many participate in daytime programmes in the community to keep them identified with the settings where they will soon be living. The court-ordered psychiatric unit at BPHCC first opened in August 1978. For its first six years (1978–84), the average length of stay at BPHCC was three years. Over the next six years (1984–89), it declined to two years. During the last six years (1990–96), the average length of stay has been only one year. This too demonstrates the natural progression occurring with the advent of more community support and better psychotropic drugs, particularly clozaril.

Involuntary in-patient days at the state hospital dropped from 5600/

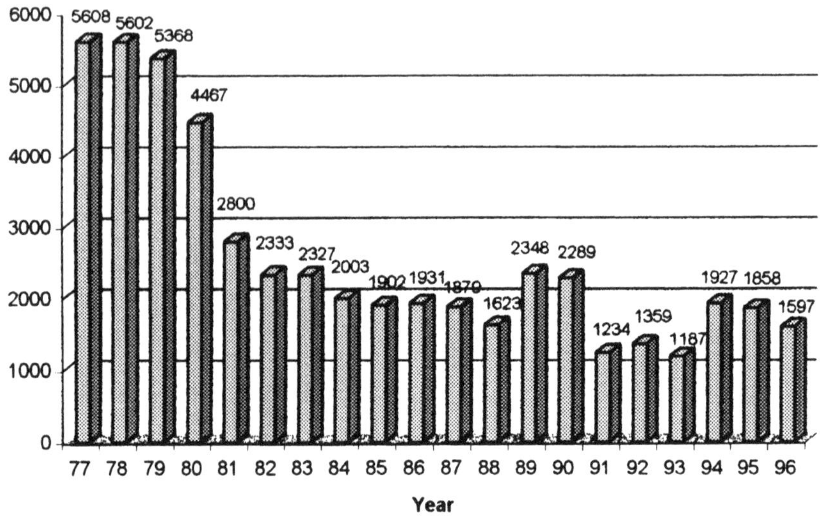

FIG. 8.3. Acute adult in-patient days. State hospital: 1977–1996.

year in the late 1970s to around 1500 in recent years (see Fig 8.3 above). This was accomplished by designating responsibilities in existing programmes and adding more alternative community programmes, all of which provided for additional responsible and effective community-based alternatives. This stability has been achieved even though funding increases have not been commensurate with higher service demands. Most involuntary in-patient admissions are for clients who are not connected to the treatment system for a variety of reasons. A five-year review of admissions revealed over 70% of the admissions to the state hospital were first-time admissions for people who had few or no service connections with the contracted system. The implication here is that a more mature system of care allows for proactivity with service connected clients and hence minimises involuntary hospitalisations or provides brief voluntary hospitalisations in community hospitals. However, there will always be persons new to the system for whom an emergency response is required—a source of unpredictability.

Psychotherapy/psychotropics. Service progression: from long-term psychotherapy to short-term, solution-focused therapy and group approaches. Long-term psychotherapy has almost been eliminated within the Madison Model in favour of reaching more people through short-term, solution focused therapy. Multiple agencies are working co-operatively to provide group therapy—a key component in this effort. Therapy groups exist to deal with such varied issues as depression, parenting, divorce, stress, learning assertiveness, surviving sexual abuse, and support for living in public housing and release from jail. Some of the groups are provided directly in the neighbourhoods where participants reside. A total of 547 people received these services in 1996 with a high degree of satisfaction reported.

Day services. Service progression: from a traditional day treatment psychotherapy emphasis to a supported employment and full-time independent employment focus. Yahara House is the primary day programme providing Level I services to over 200 people during the course of the year. While not offering the level of staff intensity and outreach assertiveness available in a CSP, Yahara House is pro-active in many instances and also uses peer supports. It is patterned after the Fountain House model and offers user-friendly and supportive services to all members who come to the house 365 days of the year. Yahara House was recently relocated to a renovated historic building near Lake Mendota whose personal charm and decor enhance its supportive milieu. It offers members a variety of groups in which to participate. Transitional employment programmes provide paid work for 40% or 83 members. There is medication dispensing and "medication groups" for many members. All members receive case management services. Meals are provided on-site in the Cafe Yahara located on the third floor. A retail store called Hidden Treasures provides work activity for

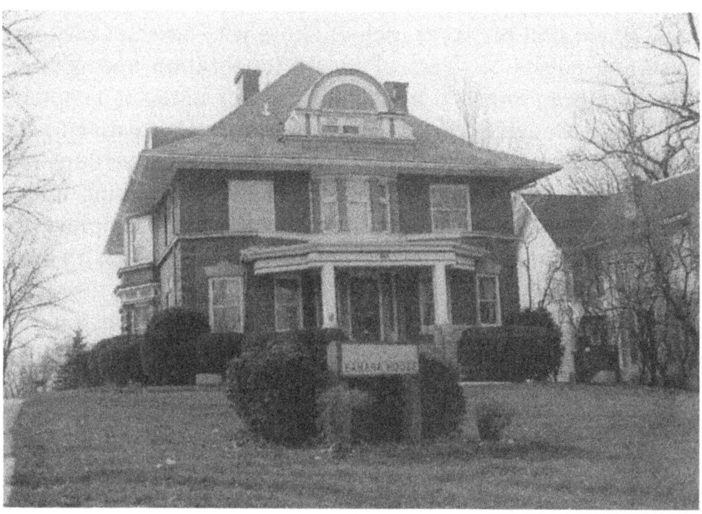

FIG. 8.4. Yahara House—A day services program.

members at another site and benefits the community at large. The programme also offers quality congregate living through its Stein and Perry Street apartment complexes (which are federal HUD-funded facilities). Staff and peer support are hallmarks of this programme. Many different work groups and several consumer self-help groups (Recovery, Inc., Alcoholics Anonymous and Narcotics Anonymous) offer ongoing opportunities for self-improvement.

Work services. Service progression: from sheltered workshops in segregated sites to supported employment in natural work sites integrated into the community. It is little wonder that gainful work has become an important treatment outcome for mental health clients. Sheltered workshops are 'out' and competitive employment in natural community settings is 'in'. Make-work has been replaced with work based on interests and on abilities in integrated community sites. Demeaning assembly-line tasks in segregated sites reinforced daydreaming which magnified symptoms. Mental health clients generally do not have to prove themselves based on earlier work performance in order to move on incrementally to more challenging work. The employer—rather than a job coach—is often the primary supervisor. Work is being incorporated into existing treatment programmes like the CSPs and Yahara House thus eliminating the need for clients to have to go through yet another programme to enter the work force. Symptom stabilisation, the single most significant factor interfering with work for mental health clients, is better managed through newer psychotropics with fewer adverse side-effects. When symptoms intensify, alternate plans are developed and implemented as needed.

The new generation of clients include those who have never experienced the devastating effects of years of institutionalisation and whose socialisation has not been impeded by the dependency-inducing hospital environment. With reasonable work incentives and better treatment, they are more ready to embrace the concept of work. Recent innovations reinforce their entry into employment, such as payment for training and higher education, which assist with both developing gainful employment and maintaining ongoing benefits (government checks and health insurance benefits).

Approximately 17% of our mental health clients perform some level of significant competitive employment and a few clients have left the security of government cheques to be on their own. The number of clients in paid employment has risen from 196 in 1991 to 257 in 1996, and their recent mean annual income was $6090.

Court-related involuntary process

The involuntary system is one of the most confusing and least understood aspects of the adult mental health system. Corporation Counsel and court-related experts have been essential to a properly working system. Knowing who to call and under what circumstances are also critical elements. In every community of the state, attorneys, the courts, law enforcement personnel, and mental health professionals have developed their own community practices based on their interpretations of the state standards for involuntary commitment. The breakdown of involuntary services for 1996 included a total of 373 persons under involuntary findings or 24% of all persons (with a serious and persistent mental illness) receiving services which included the following: 119 people under civil commitments, 75 under settlement agreements, 158 in protective services/placements, and 21 conditionally released (forensic clients). In addition to the number of persons under involuntary findings in any given year, there are others who have as a condition of their probation or parole status the taking of psychotropic medications. For these people, non-compliance can lead to placement in the Dane County Public Protection and Safety Building (jail), where mental health services are provided in an internally secure environment.

THE ROLE OF USERS IN THE SYSTEM

The role of users in our system parallels the development of the county public adult mental health system dating back to the early 1970s. The earliest user support groups prior to the development of community-based services were ex-patient groups concerned with their release from long-term in-patient stays. Their focus was to support each other and to combat professionals, for either blame or alleged abuses.

From the early activists we have evolved from adversarial to a more constructive relationship. This marked change in philosophy is evidenced by the difference in name: the first consumer organisation was called Network Against Psychiatric Assault (NAPA) while the current organisation is called Psychiatric Reform Through Education, Visionary Action and Informed Leadership (PREVAIL). Over the last 17 years, consumers and professionals have been working more effectively together in advocacy, support, and public education activities.

Today there are approximately 17 consumer focused groups, organisations and programmes that either operate within the county contracted adult system or are independent and run solely by consumers. Within the contracted system consumer involvement varies by the programme. Yahara House reflects the highest level of consumer involvement with peer support groups and staff and consumers working together on all aspects of programming. Peer Connection is the only consumer-operated, private, non-profit programme that is under contract with the county. This programme provides peer support via phone and has developed an excellent training manual for the consumer providing this service.

Consumers participate on boards and committees at all levels including hiring committees at the Mental Health Centre of Dane County. Consumers are encouraged to participate in many of the ongoing system coordination meetings and training events. Occasionally, consumers will present their own training on issues and topics where they think professionals are responding inadequately. One of the most recent consumer directed training sessions was in relation to helping professionals understand why persons with borderline personality disorders self-abuse and how better to respond to those behaviours. Consumers, staff, and representatives from the Alliance for the Mentally Ill frequently work together on public education through all forms of media. We also work together to educate local neighbourhoods to combat 'NIMBY' (Not In My Back Yard) when siting group homes.

Consumers are hired within almost all of the programmes but primarily work in staff supported housing programmes. They also work as case aides, perform janitorial and house-keeping functions within mental health programmes, and in some instances are case managers. Paid peer support is arranged through the Emergency Services Unit. The data on consumers in paid work outside the contracted system has been stated previously. Consumers are encouraged to, and do, file grievances most of which are resolved within the programmes in which they originated. If satisfaction is not achieved at the programme level it can be appealed to the county and the state. Consumers and staff mutually participate in the treatment planning, evaluation of the plan, and ongoing refinements in the plan. As evidence of the participation in this process consumers sign off on the agreed plan which is incorporated into the clinical record.

Role of the Alliance of the Mentally Ill

In September 1979 the Alliance for the Mentally Ill (AMI) of Dane County, Wisconsin, hosted the first national conference of families who have a member with a serious mental illness. The thrust of the conference was to ascertain whether persons—primarily families of persons with mental illness—were interested in forming a national alliance to work on behalf of persons with mental illnesses. Those in attendance emphatically agreed that the need for a 'family' alliance was essential. Thus during the weekend, the structure and goals of the organisation were established, along with a steering committee to guide the development of what is now the National Alliance for the Mentally Ill (NAMI). The organisations exist to advocate, educate and provide support. At this time, NAMI has over 1000 affiliates and 150,000 members. The NAMI, among many projects, is currently actively involved in a five-year anti-stigma campaign to end discrimination against persons with the brain disorders termed 'mental illnesses'.

FUTURE CHALLENGES

In the next 10 years we will continue to keep the focus of our treatment on the community. The emphasis for the public sector will continue to be on providing services to people with the most severe psychiatric disorders, and managed care organisations will be treating those who require more limited mental health interventions. As we learned at the October 1997 Mental Health in the City Conference in London, there is significant in-migration occurring into the cities and many of these people are experiencing a high level of service needs.

The most significant changes that we will be experiencing over the next decade are likely to be:

Managed care. Managed care is rapidly becoming the predominant manner in which health care services are being provided in this country. Perhaps as early as the middle of 1999, we may be implementing a managed care pilot through the state to provide a primary care model for persons who are currently receiving Medical Assistance due to their mental health disabilities. In addition to the incorporation of primary care, substance abuse treatment will also be integrated into the mental health services. There will be a single entry point into the system along with a sum certain (capitation) amount of money available. As in many of the other cities that presented at the conference, the primary care physicians will play a significant role in the delivery of mental health services with back-up being provided through our existing mental health system. Hopefully more people will have better access to psychotropics and talk therapies through this model.

Employment. At least 50% of the people should be involved in paid work in natural sites working half time and making more than the minimum wage which is currently $5.15 per hour. The state and federal government will provide more incentives for people to work by allowing for the continuation of their health benefits (Medical Assistance) while working.

In-patient. Even though the number of people who have the most severe psychiatric disorders will increase from the current level of 1537 to 2850 during this time, hospitalisations will continue to be minimised because of early symptom exacerbation detection, better psychotropics, and an even broader array of community-based alternatives. Instead of 16% of the budget going to pay for in-patient services, less than 10% will be realised by the end of the next decade, excluding people with mental health diagnoses needing 24-hour nursing home care due to their physical disabilities. One of the two state hospitals will no longer accept involuntary acute admissions, and for the first time, the county may have to operate its own speciality hospital for these people. The average length of stay (which has been constant during the past 10 years), of 15 days for involuntary admissions and 5–6 days for voluntary admissions will remain about the same.

Role of emergency services unit. This unit will continue to be the gatekeeper for in-patient services monitoring all in-patient episodes, arranging aftercare placements, and following people who are under civil commitments. While the Crisis Home programme will be expanded (currently there are nine beds), any responsible in-patient alternative will be administered through this unit. Crisis will be the entry point for many new people coming into the system.

Involuntary services. Approximately 24% of the 1537 people with the most serious psychiatric disorders are receiving some level of involuntary services at this time, many of which require the taking of psychotropic medications as prescribed. This percentage of involuntary treatment will remain about the same over the next decade. However, more of the legal findings will be for limited guardianships, meaning the person will be found incompetent due to their lack of insight into their mental illness and understanding the effectiveness of the psychotropic medication in controlling their symptoms. A guardian will then be appointed to oversee the taking of medications as prescribed.

Expansion of all of the existing services. The service stratification will remain similar with almost one-third of the people receiving community support through comprehensive assertive outreach teams. The majority of the people will be receiving level II programming as defined in this chapter, and the remaining people will receive level III services—meeting basic needs and attempting to get them connected with mental health treatment over time.

Housing. Over 90% of the consumers will be living independently in scattered site housing. A small array of supervised living arrangements will continue to be transitional.

Role of the consumer. More users will be working as a part of the mental health service delivery system and in other natural work sites in the community. They will be integrated into all aspects of the decision making process, extending their roles on current hiring committees and planning processes. Quality of life issues will be the most important evaluation outcome measurements and they will be well quantified.

CONCLUSION

The chapter closes with the critique provided by a mental health client following his reading of this preliminary report. Mr Edward Erwin has been a long-time member of Yahara House. It is reproduced below with his permission.

> 'Dignity of risk' is held up as a primary option for consumers. More importantly, it is a theme for management in an extremely responsible manner. The sense of values guiding decision making resulted in a system to which many owe much. I have been, and continue to be, a part of this wonderful 'mortal system'. Its touch is something grown into it, and its caring too often taken for granted, even by myself.
>
> I was struck by the sentences: 'All of the services are coordinated by case managers with centrally defined responsibilities (functions). This allows for flexibility and change in an orderly fashion.' I have felt the truth of this more than I have known it in these many, many years. My own and my peers' internal and external lives fit into the motion of our environment. It is our way of life. And we too often just live through rather than with these policies through levels of response to our own actions and those of others.
>
> It is impossible to sever oneself from a bureaucracy to which one is medically bound. It is also impossible for me to not look upon it as part of my own plans. Having passed through the system so far, I have my own questions as much as the mental health system does. Where to from here? My only comment, based on seeing its evolution, is this: I have confidence.

REFERENCES

Frey, J.L. (1994). Long term support: The critical element to sustaining competitive employment: Where do we begin? *Psychosocial Rehabilitation Journal*, *17*, 126–133.

Fried, C. (1996). Best places to live in America. *Money*, *25*, 66–73.

Industry Profile. (1988). Program of assertive community treatment. *Open Minds, 1*, 2.
Mosher, L. & Burti, L. (1989). An integrated system: Dane County, Wisconsin. *Community Mental Health: Principles and Practice*. New York: W.W. Norton and Company.
Stein, L.I., Diamond, R.J., & Factor, R.M. (1992). A system approach to the care of persons with schizophrenia (pp 213–246). *Handbook of Schizophrenia, Psychosocial Therapies*. Amsterdam: Elsevier Science.
Stein, L.I., Test, M.A., & Marx A. (1975). Alternative to the hospital: a Controlled Study. *American Journal of Psychiatry, 132*, 417–422.
Stein, L.I. & Test, M.A. (1980). Alternative to mental hospital treatment, III: Social cost. *Archives of General Psychiatry, 37*, 409–412.
Stein, L.I. & Test, M.A. (1980). Alternative to mental hospital treatment, I: Conceptual model, treatment program, and clinical evaluation. *Archives of General Psychiatry, 37*, 392–397.
Test, M.A. & Stein, L.I. (1978). Training in community living: research design and results. In L. Stein & M.A. Test (Eds), *Alternatives to Mental Hospital Treatment* (pp 57–74). New York: Plenum.
Thompson, K.S., Griffith, E.H., & Philip, J.L. (1990). A historical review of the Madison Model of community care. *Hospital and Community Psychiatry, 41*, 625–634.
Torrey, E.F. & Wolfe, S.M. (1986). *Care of the Seriously Mentally Ill: a Rating of State Programs* (p. 48). Washington, DC: Public Citizen Health Research Group.
Weisbrod, B.A., Test, M.A., & Stein, L.I. (1980). Alternative to mental hospital treatment, II: Economic benefit-cost analysis. *Archives of General Psychiatry, 37*, 400–405.

CHAPTER NINE

City of Porto Alegre, Brazil: The Brazilian concept of quality of life

Dinarte A.P. Ballester and Ana Cristina Tietzmann
Fundação Faculdade Federal de Ciências Médicas de Porto Alegre, RS Brazil
Ariadne Runte Geidel and Patricia Zillmer
Escola Especial Municipal Luis Francisco Lucena Borges, RS Brazil
Maria de Fátima Fischer and Miriam Dias
Secretaria Municipal de Saúde, RS Brazil
Ellis D'Arrigo Busnello
Fundação Faculdade Federal de Ciências Médicas de Porto Alegre, RS Brazil

THE CITY AND ITS HISTORY

In 1740, Jerônimo de Ornelas from Portugal received the definitive title to the lands, and moved to the property with his whole family, relatives and employees, and in 1772 the settlement was officially founded and received the name of Our Lady Mother of God of Porto Alegre. In 1773 the central government of Brazil, as part of the Kingdom of Portugal, made Porto Alegre the capital city of Rio Grande do Sul. Urbanisation began and the main buildings were erected. Between 1860 and 1886 the city grew faster as industry developed. During this period several improvements occurred, such as the inauguration of the Waterworks Company to supply drinking water to the whole population, inauguration of public transport, the telegraph station, the City Council Building, Public Library and São Pedro Psychiatric Hospital, as well as the Telephone Union. The Republic was proclaimed in Brazil in 1889, and enthusiastically received by the inhabitants of Porto Alegre.

The city of Porto Alegre entered the 20th century with a large population and economically developed. Among the urban facilities were public transport, water and wastewater services, telephones, elementary and secondary schools and institutions of higher education, active trade, developing industries, and a numerous, varied press.

PORTO ALEGRE TODAY

Demographic structure

The conjunction of changes in demographic pattern and urbanisation at the end of this century has caused profound structural changes which will have a strong impact on the future of social and economic development in Brazil. The speedy urbanisation process that occurred between the years of 1940 and 1980 led to a significant reduction in the rural population and in towns with less than 20,000 inhabitants. The population in these areas dropped from 85% to 46%, while the remainder drifted to urban areas. Large cities with more than half a million population accounted for 32% of the population. Beginning in the 1980s, this process underwent a reversal, involving a significant reduction in urban population growth rate and deceleration of the population concentration in the large cities. Thus, the core cities of metropolitan areas such as Porto Alegre presented a reduction in their annual growth rates during the 1970s and 1980s, growing less than their metropolitan regions. In Porto Alegre the annual growth rate which had been 2.4% between 1970 and 1980 became 1.1% between 1980 and 1991.

The city of Porto Alegre has a total area of 471 km^2, consisting of a continental part of 428 km^2 and the Islands, 43 km^2. The Porto Alegre population, after the county boundaries with Viamão changed in 1992, is 1.25 million inhabitants, with a demographic density of 2.6 inhabitants/km^2. The age structure of the population is that 27% of the population are below the age of 15, two-thirds are between 15 and 64, and the remaining 6.6% above 65 years old. The fact that the school age population is growing at an increasingly smaller rate, which will extend to the end of the century, allows a slower expansion of the education system. The investment in education should be made not by increasing the physical facilities but mainly by raising the quality of teaching in Brazilian schools. The Brazilian education system is generally considered very weak, and requires a leap forward in quality to overcome the deficiencies found in elementary and secondary schools. The rising number of aged in the population forecast by all demographic studies could worsen the problem of unassisted senior citizens that already occurs in Brazil. The aged will find it harder to survive since they will belong to smaller and smaller families, due to the sharp decrease in fertility which has occurred in Brazil. This sector of the population has trouble finding shelter and help from children and close relatives, and represents a difficult social problem.

Economic aspects

The Participative budget. This budget was adopted to prepare the Plan of Investments to be made in the city with the participation of the population. It is a public form of civil power, independent of the government. It allows citizens to participate in municipal government and make decisions about the budget as a whole. This means greater democracy, since the population participates in local government. The city is divided into 16 regions, in each of which meetings are held to discuss priorities and elect councillors. Meetings since 1994 have addressed five main themes: transportation; economic development and taxation; city organisation and urban development; health and welfare; and education, culture, and leisure. Thus, it is easy to participate: all it takes is that citizens attend the meetings which are always announced by the neighbourhood associations and in the press. Meetings are also held in the communities to choose local priorities: sanitation, paving, housing, health, education, and so on.

At the intermediate meetings more delegates may be elected, considering the people present at the meeting with the highest quorum, and using the same criteria as for the election of delegates during the first round. Then the Forum of Delegates is completed in each of the regions and themes. Resources to be invested in the city are apportioned according to the following criteria, since the regions are unequal: lack of a service or urban infrastructure in the region, and size of the total population. These criteria receive scores and weights, which make it possible to set up a grid with all regions and the investments to be made in them.

Economic sectors. Porto Alegre county has three main economic sectors: agriculture and animal husbandry, industry, services and trade. In 1992, the municipal per capita income was US$5307.

Approximately 30% of the territory of the capital is described as rural, over half of it with farming potential. The main agricultural products in the county are peaches, oranges, husk rice, manioc, and tomatoes. Besides agriculture there are also animal husbandry activities with poultry, pigs, cows and sheep, as well as dairy products. However, only 0.5% of the municipal work force is employed in the agricultural sector.

The manufacturing industry has a small share in jobs in Porto Alegre, with 11.0% of the overall work force (PMPA, 1996). Manufacturing can be divided into two approximately equal segments: modern industry (such as metallurgy, mechanics, electronics, rubber, chemistry, plastics, and pharmaceuticals) and traditional industry (such as furniture and wood products, arts and crafts, textiles, clothing, footwear, foodstuffs, glass, ceramics, building materials, and printing).

Finally, services account for 16% of the total jobs, and services account for the remainder of the workforce.

Jobs and income. The picture of macroeconomic instability in the Brazilian economy since the beginning of the 1980s, with a drop in the rate of investments, a fall in manufacturing in a context of economic expansion has had a negative impact on the world of labour, worsening the already dramatic social inequalities in Brazil. This has led to the establishment of employment promotion policies and compensatory social policies.

Income distribution is concentrated in the same way as in the rest of the country, although Porto Alegre's Gini index, 0.57 in 1991, is lower as compared with other Brazilian cities. The Gini index measures income inequality, and its limit values are 0 and 1. In other words, maximum inequality would attain index 1, whereas at 0 all inhabitants would have the same income.

Profile of the economically active population

The active age population (AAP) consisted of just over 1 million persons in 1993, corresponding to 83% of the people living in the county that year. Females predominate in this population, representing 54% of this group. Most of those in the AAP (84.,6%) were Caucasian. The heads of households constituted 36% of the AAP, while spouses represented 24.2% and children 31% of the total. The economically active population (EAP) of Porto Alegre in 1993 was 601,000 persons, of whom 89% had an occupation, and the other 11% were unemployed or looking for work.

Individuals in the 18–24 year age group and those 25–39 had the most significant rates of participation in employment (72% and 81%, respectively), while among persons 40 years old and over, only half (50.6%) were economically active. Caucasian individuals had a slightly lower rate of participation in the labour market than non-Caucasians (56% *vs* 59%).

Distribution of income. Only about 12.1% of the population earned below the recommended minimum wage, and 19% earned between 5 and 10 times the minimum wage, with a further 18% earning more than 10 times the minimum wage. However, even greater inequalities are found in other Brazilian cities.

Absolute poverty line in Porto Alegre. The 1990s have been marked by renewed interest on the part of international agencies such as UNO and the World Bank in the reduction of absolute poverty. In several countries, of which Brazil is a clear example, the benefits of economic growth have not been extended to the population as a whole. Thus, contrasts in levels of income and living conditions between the poor and non-poor persist and continue to rise, especially in the urban areas where the phenomenon is more visible. Approximately one-third of a million individuals, or 92,000 families, were below the absolute poverty line in Porto Alegre in 1993. The profile of the poor population indicates that poor families are larger, on average (3.9 individuals as compared with 3.1 in other families), with predominance of younger people (47.3% of the poor individuals are aged up to 17, while 29.7% of the non-poor are in this age range). Children and non-Caucasians are also over-represented, and the level of formal schooling is low among poor people.

Housing, basic sanitation and transport

According to the 1991 census, in Porto Alegre there are 325,461 domiciles with 4 or more rooms, representing 85.7% of the total number of homes. This indicates a reasonable degree of comfort in the home for most of the population, taking into account that there are, on average, 3.29 residents per domicile and 5.80 rooms per home. In 1996, 99% of the Porto Alegre population had drinking water supplied inside their homes, and 78% had sanitary installations connected to the general sewage network. Garbage collection in Porto Alegre covers all homes, after Project 'Garbage Collection in Areas Difficult to Approach' was implemented in 1990. Selective domestic garbage collection, implemented in the County in 1990, covers 97% of the city neighbourhoods, and also provides income for over 250 people who survive directly from the sale of materials obtained in the selective garbage collection (PMPA,1996). Seventy-eight percent of the road system of Porto Alegre is paved. The housing situation of the low income population is an historical problem in Brazil. The population living in sub-normal domiciles, also called 'favelas', grew from 3.1% to 4.2% of the Brazilian counties during the 1980s. In the Porto Alegre Metropolitan Region, in 1991, there were 105 favelas, with 31,781 homes. More recent estimates performed by the Municipal Department of Housing indicate that there are 289 favelas, with 20.4% of the city's population, in 67,470 domiciles (PMPA, 1997).

Education

The situation regarding education in Brazil, despite considerable recent improvements, is still considered very poor as compared, for instance, with that of the other seven richest countries of Latin America, in which the average schooling of the population is 6.9 years, whereas in Brazil it is around 4 years. This factor has great weight since it conditions the quality of the work force which, in turn, is associated with the level of formal education and influences the income from work. The literacy rate in the urban area was 95%, and 80% in the rural area. There are four municipal special schools for children with special educational needs, as well as other private schools.

Culture, leisure and sports

The County of Porto Alegre has 10 universities or colleges, 38 buildings which have been registered as National Heritage, 26 libraries, 24 museums, 12 theatres, 39 art galleries, and 22 auditoriums.

There are 505 public squares with a mean area of 7237 square metres and 8 parks in the public domain, comprising 18.19 square kilometres. Furthermore it keeps 17 municipal football fields and 34 recreation units with multisports pitches, football fields, bowling, volleyball, basketball, indoor football, athletics, and tennis.

HEALTH

Life expectancy and low birth weight babies

Life expectancy at birth during the three-year period from 1979 to 1981 was 64 for males and 74 for females, a figure lower than that for the most recent estimate—76.6yrs. An assessment of the percentages of low birth weight (less than 2500g) showed an increase in the last few years, from 8.9 in 1992 to 9.4 in 1995. This figure is intermediate between that for developed countries such as Sweden (4%), and developing countries like India (30%). In Porto Alegre, low weight related to prematurity constituted 52% of the cases and intrauterine malnutrition 48%.

Health policies in Brazil and Porto Alegre

Health in Brazil is organised under the form of the Unified Health System (*Sistema Único de Saúde, SUS*), according to which health is the right of the citizen and the duty of the state, independent of any contribution paid to social security. The annual expenditure on health is $222 per person per year.

The principles of SUS are universal health care coverage; full, broad health care; equality, that is all have the right to health, taking into account social inequalities, social justice and income redistribution; decentralisation of health actions, so that the counties alone are in charge of system management; and community participation in the formulation of strategies, inspection, and social control of health actions, through the health conferences and health councils, at the national, state, and municipal levels. They are constituted by representatives of managers, service providers, health care workers, and the population of health service users. The participation of the community (users) should have parity with the other segments.

The SUS is a public system funded by the government (federal, state and municipal), with resources from the social contributions of employers and employees (based on the payroll), invoicing and profit of companies, revenue from prognostic competitions (lotteries), public budgets, rates, and taxes.

Care for the population is provided via government services and private services which have an agreement or a contract, the latter to complement the government service network. Besides the SUS service network, there is a broad range of private health services and different levels of complexity, which the population can access via private health plans or direct payment.

In Brazil, in the last decades, the public health services have been scrapped and great privileges were bestowed on private health services. The care supplied by these services is known to be rather inaccessible and expensive. More sophisticated diagnostic and therapeutic resources are used to excess in some cases, although they are unattainable for most of the population at times when they would be essential. Moreover, users are often obliged to pay for procedures 'on the side', even though they are funding the public health services by paying direct and indirect taxes.

The low capacity of public out-patient care units to solve problems, both in Porto Alegre and in the metropolitan region generates demands which wind up in the hospital emergency services, and affect the ability of these services to care for real emergencies. According to assessments by the emergency service of the Hospital de Clínicas de Porto Alegre, 75% of the cases seen would be simple visits to the doctor.

The County of Porto Alegre took over the running of the health system alone in August 1996, by transferring financial, political and administrative management as well as personnel, equipment (physical structures), actions, and services from the federal and state government levels to the counties.

The population has difficulty in obtaining hospital beds, since approximately 48% of the hospital admissions are people from the interior of the state. For some specific diseases such as heart, cancer and AIDS there is a lack of beds. The city administration took over 51 state and federal health units which were in a bad condition, and over 1500 employees, besides the areas that were insufficient. This was in addition to 15 other units, that the city administration was already maintaining. The administration has been working to change this profile, giving 14% of its budget to health. Of this total, 48% are consumed by the Hospital de Pronto Socorro (the city emergency hospital) to which people come from all over the state.

A computerised central station is being implemented to make appointments for visits and specialised exams to ensure that everyone has equal right of access to specialised care. The purpose of the central station is to organise the service and identify areas with a higher demand and lack of specialists; in this system the health unit makes the appointments. In 1996, the Municipal Department of Health set up 24 teams of the Family Health Project (*PSF-Projeto de Saúde da Família*) in deprived areas without health care. These sites were defined by the community in the regional fora of Participative budget delegates, local health councils, and approved by the Municipal Health Council. The present situation is a major challenge to be faced in order to organise and manage services for the best care of the population.

Mental health policy in Porto Alegre

The first milestone of public mental health care occurred when psychiatric hospitals were created at the end of the last century. Hospital Psiquiátrico São Pedro, founded in 1884, was the first specialised service for the care of mental patients. Over the years conditions deteriorated because of overcrowding, with over 5000 patients in the 1960s, at the same time as mental health expenditures were concentrated on this hospital.

Beginning in the 1970s, the state expanded mental health services. In contrast to the rest of Brazil, the state of Rio Grande do Sul established mental health out-patient clinics at the Sanitary Units, and installed the Centre for Agricultural Rehabilitation at Colonia Itapuã. A specialised out-patient clinic was also set up, the Central de Psiquiatria, unconnected with the general health services.

The private services network under agreements with the public system, expanded in the state interior and the capital, and alternative services were set up, including day hospitals, sheltered housing, and therapeutic communities. At the same time, the general living conditions among the population at large became worse due to the economic policy of the military dictatorship. At the end of the 1970s, the state mental health guidelines aimed at dehospitalisation, sectorisation, preventive work, and making use of local resources and general health services.

Beginning in the 1980s, priorities and programmes were defined based on the World Health Organization proposal for primary health care. These health actions had a limited effect due to insufficient investment of resources and discontinuity caused by changes in public administration. The changes in Brazil's health policy, especially after the 1988 Constitution, influenced the lines of mental health care. Similarly, the National Conferences on Mental Health, in 1987 and 1991, caused major changes in legislation.

In the state of Rio Grande do Sul, the Law of Psychiatric Reform was passed in 1992, legitimising the need to reorganise mental health care. The Law determines that beds in psychiatric hospitals will be progressively replaced by a complete mental health care system. It determines rules to protect people suffering from psychiatric problems, especially from compulsory psychiatric hospitalisation. These changes are to come about by means of a single management for the different services and their organisations in districts, respecting universal need for health, and the principles of equality and user participation.

Principles and guidelines for the Mental Health Service

The full mental health care services should:

1. Be constituted by interdisciplinary teams.
2. Allow the subjects to maintain or construct their own social and cultural bonds.
3. Receive all those who seek the services, without any distinction which might lead to exclusion and segregation.
4. Avoid social isolation and complete permanent invalidity caused by prolonged hospitalisation, especially in psychiatric hospitals.
5. Permanently question the health workers as to their daily practice and relationships established with the public institution, the team, the users, and the community.
6. Organise the services in order to make them available for care and/or listening.
7. Identify the form of community organisation, cultural and social patterns, potential and manifest forms of expression.
8. Question the belief that links mental disease directly to disability.
9. Establish channels of communication for users to plan and assess the functioning of the services.
10. Treat persons as to their unique aspects, acknowledging each one's critical capacity and choice of mode of treatment appropriate to their needs, as well as their evaluation of it.
11. Acknowledge that each person knows his symptoms, disease, development capacity, life, and plans.
12. The therapeutic plan should take into account the new meaning and/or construction of life projects of each individual, shared socially (family, friends, neighbours, community, institutions).
13. Respect the mental patients as citizens, acknowledging the truth in their discourse.
14. Acknowledge mental patients as citizens beyond what the diagnosis defines as their disease.
15. Avoid the reductionism of the biological paradigm incorporating the contributions of the different fields of knowledge, such as anthropology, psycho-analysis, sociology.

16. Develop projects to provide full attention to mental health among the population currently living on the streets right where they are, respecting the values and behavioural patterns constituted based on this reality.

This whole process of change is permeated by the principle of building up citizenship which assumes that there are self-organisation processes favouring expression, participation, and the constitution of the identity of an individual in his relationship with the world and his fellow men.

The Municipal Mental Health Plan

The Municipal Mental Health Plan organises the public services respecting the specificities of each health district (approximately 100,000 people). The health teams at each health unit must be able to respond to the mental health demands integrated with the other health actions. Mental health teams should be part of more complex general services and Centres of Integrated Mental Health Care (CAIS mental centres) to attend to more complex levels of care. The Therapeutic and Income Generation Workshops may be linked to the CAIS mental centres and sheltered housing distributed throughout the districts where there is a specific demand for this type of service. Moreover, services are to be established for emergencies as well as beds for admission to general hospitals.

For each 100,000 population at risk, there are 24.3 psychiatrists, 37.9 acute beds, 48 chronic beds, 5.4 nurses with University degrees, and 45.6 nursing auxiliaries.

Health teams in general services

The health care provided by interdisciplinary teams is permeated by mental health actions since it may foster the expression of feelings on the part of a person who comes to the service for any procedure and take comprehensive care of the individual. Therefore, every health worker can be a mental health agent. In order to do so it is necessary to train, supervise and provide continued education for these professionals.

The mental health team

This team must respond to the demands referred to them by the other health services in the district, supervise and advise the work performed by the other units, and interact with CAIS mental center. This is the team which must resist the trend to centralisation of health actions at hospitals and work with the institutions and the organised community of the area it covers, on social processes that generate a risk of psychiatric illness.

The team should consist of a psychologist, psychiatrist, psychiatric nurse, and social worker. It only exists in places where the need is greater due to higher demographic density, demand, and/or lack of resources to provide welfare.

Centres of Integrated Mental Health Care (CAIS mental centres)

In the original proposal, this should be characterised as a specialised service with immediate availability and beds for brief hospital stays and observation, functioning 24 hours a day as a specialised place of reference for each district. The team should consist of psychologists, social workers, psychiatrists, therapeutic 'friend', nursing aides, nurse, occupational therapist, psychological health teacher, physical education teacher and audiologist.

Currently, there are only two CAIS mental centres providing out-patient care, day care centre and therapeutic workshops. The day care centre receives patients who have been discharged from psychiatric hospitals or are in crisis and remain under treatment during the daytime. The therapeutic workshops are coordinated by occupational therapists.

Sheltered workshops

The purpose of the workshops is to develop activities of socialisation, professional education, leisure and art, for patients referred by health teams and open to the community at large. They are to integrate the mental health service users in the community to which they belong. In order to function they must integrate with the Department of Health, Education, Culture, Foundation of Social and Community Education, and other agencies of organised civil society. The CAIS mental centre team is to coordinate the work developed together with professionals from specific fields such as: figurative arts, ceramics, music, dancing, handicrafts. The sheltered workshop should foster the establishment of work cooperatives depending on how the activities in these workshops continue to develop.

Sheltered housing

The Sheltered Housing Project offers a concrete opportunity to put aside the asylum model for patients who have become institutionalised, without any real prospects of entering or re-entering society. A more detailed description of the project is given below under 'Creating new social structures'.

Mental health emergencies

The goal to be achieved is integration with the general emergency services of the emergency hospitals and/or general hospitals in the districts, with a team constituted by nurses, general practitioner, psychiatrists, neurologists, psychologist, social worker, and nursing aides. Currently emergency care for the whole city is provided at the 'Psychiatric Central' only during the daytime and is not sufficient to satisfy demand. Some cases are seen in the admissions services of psychiatric hospitals.

The role of the general hospital mental health unit

The goal of the mental health units of general hospitals should be short hospital stays, receiving patients referred by public and/or extra-hospital university services, and developing multi-professional therapeutic activities in order to achieve remission of the symptoms and/or signs which caused hospitalisation. It should be pointed out that for this purpose it is necessary to have a daily programme of therapeutic activities, besides medication and family group involvement in this programme.

The team should provide care for the other units of the hospital when psychiatric events occur and for psychoprophylactic activities. The multi-professional team should promote systematic contacts with the health service network in its district, creating a system of reference and counter-reference. The number of psychiatric beds available in general hospital should obey the ruling of the Ministry of Health in which 10% of the bed capacity is to be provided for psychiatric care, up to a maximum of 30 beds per hospital.

The understanding is that the institutionalising functions of the mental hospitals and the stigma associated with them prevent them from establishing satisfactory conditions for therapeutic change. Human resources currently located at these places should be transferred to the general care network. Since mental health units in general hospitals and other community services can more effectively solve and take care of existing demands, mental hospitals will be gradually decommissioned.

PSYCHIATRIC MORBIDITY INDICATORS IN PORTO ALEGRE

According to data from the Psychiatric Morbidity Study on the Urban Population of Porto Alegre (Busnello et al., 1992), the estimated prevalence of psychiatric morbidity in the Porto Alegre population is 49%. The three most frequent diagnoses are disorders due to the use of psychoactive substances (24.6%), anxiety disorders (23%), and affective disorders

(10.7%). When the diagnosis of tobacco dependence whose prevalence was estimated as 20.1% is excluded, there is still a high estimated prevalence of mental illness of 42.7%.

Alcohol use disorders, including abuse and dependence, have an estimated prevalence of 8.8%, and in men the risk is considerably higher than in women (relative risk: 7.13). For the other psychoactive substances a population estimate of 2.5% was found. In the anxiety disorders group, the diagnosis of simple phobia has an estimated prevalence of 12.8%, with a higher risk among women (RR: 2.53). The other anxiety disorders have the

TABLE 9.1
Diagnoses and Percentage Prevalence Coefficients (Psychiatric Morbidity Study on the Urban Population of Porto Alegre)

*Disorder**	*N*	*Year Prevalence†* *(estimated) %*
General total (including smoking)	(163)	49.0
Disorder due to use of psychoactive substances		
Total	(81)	24.6
Tobacco dependence	(65)	20.1
Alcohol use disorder	(24)	8.8
Disorder due to use of other substances	(10)	2.5
Anxiety disorders		
Total	(80)	23.0
Simple phobia	(46)	12.8
Generalised anxiety	(31)	6.7
Agoraphobia	(8)	2.8
Obsessive-compulsive disorder	(7)	1.6
Social phobia	(5)	0.9
Other anxiety disorders	(3)	1.5
Panic disorders	(2)	1.1
Affective disorders		
Total	(40)	10.7
Major depression	(21)	5.7
Dysthymic disorder	(18)	4.6
Bipolar disorder	(2)	0.6
Cyclothymic disorder	(1)	0.6
Mental deficiency	(12)	4.6
Psychological factors affecting physical status	(12)	3.5
Somatoform disorders	(18)	3.2
Adjustment disorders	(5)	1.4
Organic brain diseases (dementia)	(6)	1.2
Schizophrenia	(4)	0.9
Other psychotic disorders	(1)	0.1

* Diagnostic criteria according to DSM-III.

† Population estimate adjusted by distribution of genders QMPA (Screening instrument).

No atypical bipolar, paranoia (delusional), food, factitious and impulse control disorders cases were found; psychosexual disorders were not researched.

following population estimates: generalised anxiety (6.7%), agoraphobia (2.8%), obsessive-compulsive disorder (2.6%), panic disorder (1.1%), others (1.1%). Among the affective disorders, the third most frequently observed group of diagnoses, estimates were as follows: major depression (5.7%), dysthymic disorder (4.6%), bipolar disorder (0.6%), cyclothymic disorder (0.6%). The fourth most frequent disorder referred to mental deficiency, with a population estimate of 4.6%, high as compared to data from literature (3%), which could be attributed to socio-economic conditions. Schizophrenia has an estimated prevalence of 0.9%.

Table 9.1 describes the groups of diagnoses and the percentage prevalence coefficients in the sample and estimated year prevalence in the population over 15 years old.

The estimate for the potential demand of mental disorders in Porto Alegre is higher for alcohol abuse or dependence and anxiety disorders and depression, as observed in Table 9.2.

This study was part of the Multicentred Study on Neurological and Psychiatric Morbidity in Brazilian Urban Areas which constituted the first experience in Brazil of a broad investigation of mental health in urban populations (IBGE, 1991). In Porto Alegre and in the other cities that participated in the study, São Paulo and Brasília, indexes of Global Prevalence Estimate (GPE) and of Potential Demand Estimate (PDE) of mental disorders were observed as shown in Table 9.2.

TABLE 9.2
Estimates of Psychiatric Morbidity by Diagnosis (DSM-III), in Three Metropolitan Areas. Brazil, 1990–1991

Diagnosis	*Brasilia*		*Sao Paulo*		*Porto Alegre*	
	PDE	*GPE*	*PDE*	*GPE*	*PDE*	*GPE*
Anxiety disorder	12.1	17.6	6.9	10.6	5.4	9.6
Phobic disorder	11.6	16.7	5.0	7.6	7.1	14.1
Somatodissociative disorders	5.8	8.1	1.9	2.8	2.8	4.8
Obsessive-compulsive disorders	0.5	0.7	–	–	1.2	2.1
Adjustment disorder	1.3	2.0	0.4	0.6	1.0	1.6
Depression	1.5	2.8	1.3	1.9	6.7	10.2
Mania and cyclothymia	0.3	0.4	0.2	0.3	1.0	1.1
Psychoses	0.2	0.3	0.6	0.9	2.0	2.9
Alcohol abuse/ dependence	4.7	8.0	4.3	7.6	8.7	9.2
Mental retardation	1.9	3.0	1.6	2.6	1.8	3.4
Global	34.1	50.5	19.0	31.0	33.7	42.5

The sum of global prevalence does not correspond to the sum of specific prevalences due to the presence of co-occurrence.

COMMUNITY PARTICIPATION IN THE HEALTH SYSTEM

During the military regime, financial problems accumulated and several changes became necessary. As democracy returned, the channels of participation in political decisions began to reopen, and many changes were achieved in the Brazilian health system, both due to the pressure of popular movements and the unions and to proposals of reform by congressmen. The Federal Constitution of 1988 and the Laws of the Unified Health System (1991) reformed the system, enabling the municipal sphere to exert decisive and growing influence on health policies.

Thus, from the second half of the last decade onwards the municipal sphere of government gradually became more important in the system. The committees, and then the municipal health councils had the power to plan and supervise the use of financial resources transferred from the federal sphere of government to the municipal level.

Several mechanisms were created by the 1988 Constitution to operationalise popular participation in managing the system. Previously the users had been organised in a more centralised manner in municipal or even state entities or else through workers' unions. Although these entities were better organised than other more decentralised popular movements closer to the population, such as the Community Associations in each neighbourhood or low-income area that had their roots in the community struggles for health still in the 1970s, several factors were accountable for the gradual change in the form of user participation.

Beginning with changes in the health system, Porto Alegre County gradually took over this new form of organisation and, working with the population, established the structures and form of management of this new system—the Regional Interinstitutional Health Committees (CRIS). Initially meetings were held during working hours, thus favouring the participation of representatives of health unit professionals and service suppliers, but making it difficult for the users to participate. All the same, several things were achieved, such as building new, equipped health units, especially in Porto Alegre areas where urban popular movements were stronger and better organised.

Legal changes

Several discussions were held with the executive level of government to regulate, by municipal law, the existence of the Municipal Health Council and, thus, the representations in the different regions of Porto Alegre. The Municipal Health Council of Porto Alegre passed a Complementary Law in 1992: a Deliberative Body of the Single Health System, defining as its competence:

1. To define the health priorities.
2. To establish and decide on guidelines.
3. To control the implementation of health policies.
4. To propose criteria for scheduling and financial and budget implementations.
5. To follow, assess and inspect the health services provided to the population.
6. To study and sign contracts and agreements between the public sector and private entities.
7. To define criteria on quantity and quality of health services.

The Municipal Health council is a collegiate organ constituted by representatives of the Municipal Government (Executive Power), health professionals, service providers, and users. These representatives adopt the following distribution: half the places are for user representatives, and the other places are for government representatives, service providers and health professionals. The Council is also constituted by Committees, amongst which is the Mental Health Committee.

The Mental Health Committee was established in 1992, in response to a requirement in the Psychiatric Reform Law of Rio Grande do Sul. This Committee is concerned with planning, following, inspecting, and evaluating the mental health policy in Porto Alegre, operating by delegation of the Municipal Health Council. It is constituted by representatives of the municipal, state and federal governments, professional classes related to mental health, public hospitals and hospitals working with the Unified Health System, unions, community, user and family member organisations. Some organisations are *AGAFAPE* (Schizophrenic Patients Relatives Association) and *Mental Health Forum of Rio Grande do Sul*.

Local health councils (CLS)

After the Municipal Health Council had been duly regulated, the CLS (local health councils) were organised. These were at district level, which are currently the participative forums closest to the population. The CLS are constituted by representatives of different organisations such as Associations of Inhabitants, Community Associations, Mothers' Clubs, schools, and others. Besides planning, evaluating and controlling health in the region (neighbourhoods and/or low income areas) the CLS are beginning to have the possibility of managing the financial resources they receive, based on the organisation of local managers councils. Currently, Porto Alegre is divided into 11 health districts, each district with a corresponding CLS. There is also a discrepancy in the health service network of each region or district, therefore each CLS is responsible for the social control of a different number of services.

The representatives of the various organisations that constitute the CLS meet monthly, in the evening, to provide an opportunity for the participation of the users' representatives to plan, discuss and evaluate health actions. From the beginning, coordinators were elected, responsible for organising the schedule of the meetings, the agenda according to topics presented by the group present and coordinating the meeting proper, besides representing the CLS at the Municipal Health Council (CMS).

The CLS can promote events such as local conferences, seminars and study rounds on the topics which seem relevant to the needs of the region. It is in the CLS that the most pressing needs of the population appear, and where pertinent actions are articulated for solution or referral. In democratic discussion demands are prioritised and solutions initiated.

Creating new social structures

Project Housing. The purpose of this project is to revert the trend to social isolation, strengthening ties with the family, the neighbourhood, and the community at large. Housing should be considered temporary, depending on the individuality of each person. The project includes two programmes:

1. Sheltered Housing (Boarding House) '*Nova Vida*' (New Life): this is a residence, in a public building, with a specific team to provide care (nursing aides and 'therapeutic friends') to benefit people with poor socio-economic resources. It was planned to shelter at most 20 persons with full care and connected to the CAIS mental centre. At present there are 20 persons, former inmates of psychiatric hospitals.
2. Transition House (*Casa de Transição*): it is a house connected to this programme for the purpose of developing skills in organising living and autonomy for mental patients who are psychically and economically capable of self-maintenance. The expansion of this programme includes the rental or purchase of houses or apartments

for small groups (three to four persons), who will be responsible for the daily maintenance activities of the home. The people who live in these homes will be connected to treatment at the CAIS mental centres in the workshops and helped to enter the labour market.

Special Municipal School Luís Francisco Lucena Borges. The school was founded in September 1990, and takes care of children and adolescents who present development disorders (autism, psychosis, hyperactivity) but began to receive a large number of children and adolescents who had other emotional problems associated with mental deficiency.

The School Regulations, the most important document in the school, was constructed by the school community with its four segments: parents, pupils, employees and teachers. The school community began to elect the school principal, and recently also began to manage the allotments for the school's expenditures.

Currently the school curriculum is organised in three "Formation Cycles": Basic Learning, Schooling and Becoming Independent. The curriculum seeks to prepare pupils both for working and for regular education, since the main purpose of this school is the integration of the individual into the community.

In this school there is participation by; organising groups which seek to discuss the rights of children and adolescents with development disorders, in several forums, such as through the Participative budget, the local health council, and the Municipal Mental Health Committee.

INTEGRATION BETWEEN FACULTY AND HEALTH SERVICES IN TEACHING PSYCHIATRY

Porto Alegre has three medical schools. All of them have psychiatry and mental health departments and services. We will describe the model of health care, teaching and research proposed by the Department of Psychiatry and Psychiatric Service of the *Fundação Faculdade Federal de Ciências Médicas de Porto Alegre (FFFCMPA)*, in association with the *Hospital Materno Infantil Presidente Vargas,* (HMIPV), a mother–child care hospital.

The Presidente Vargas Hospital is a specialized site of tertiary care for women and children. In a way it treats a population of women who present with problems of the fertile cycle, as well as children and adolescents of both genders, all of them described as high risk.

The Psychiatric Service was introduced in 1991, in response to the Law of Psychiatric Reform of the State of Rio Grande do Sul, which required the integration of psychiatric services to that general hospital. It includes a 25 bed in-patient unit and an out-patient clinic. At first the OP clinic provided care for the patients who had been discharged from the in-patient unit, and later to respond to the demand which has already become considerable, since the clientele sought to find the whole range of services they required in one place. Soon the Consultancy and Liaison and Community and Social Psychiatry Units were added.

The Psychiatric Department and Service actively train physicians; in the undergraduate course they develop disciplines and internships with families and in the community, the out-patient clinic and in-patient unit at the hospital. The disciplines developed are oriented to the study of human life and personal development, the doctor–patient relationship and clinical psychiatry. In order to train specialists in graduate courses, teaching is organised under the form of residency programmes. These programmes seek to contribute to train physicians and specialists providing them with knowledge of psychiatry and mental health. The academic and hospital psychiatric service that was being created adopted a programme and a structure that emphasised psychiatric and mental health practice where the biological, psychological, and social fundamentals of population care had a counterpoint in teaching and research adapted to them. Therefore, the introduction of a strong community and social component in undergraduate and graduate training was a paradigm of teaching developed since the beginning of the programmes aiming to provide future and already practising physicians with knowledge, skills and attitudes allowing good psychiatric practice by non-specialists. From its inception the service was organised in an innovative manner, establishing agreements with the newly formed community mental health services.

Several teachers in the psychiatric department sought and are seeking postgraduate training in MSc. and PhD. courses, aiming to form the teachers and researchers of the future. Research is expected to receive a strong impulse in coming years. The Head of the Psychiatric Service and Professor of the Department maintains a line of research in community and social psychiatry, extension of mental health care for populations, and social aspects and diseases. These are areas which concentrate interests that are essential to establish adequate mental health policies and to develop conventional and innovative mental health Services.

This organisation of health care, teaching and research with the common denominator of defined population interests, modifies the conventional organisation of teaching and research in mental health performed at conventional institutions of higher education. Knowledge regarding the population, the diagnosis of their health problems, and the definition of health priorities to be fulfilled, as well as the need to involve the population in their care, require innovative forms of service and the use of adequate technologies able to maintain a high quality of care which can be provided to a large number of members of the population defined.

FUTURE CHALLENGES

The care of individual mental health in a society could be considered an indicator of quality of life. Conversely, the combination of factors which determine quality of life in a collective group, whether economic, ecological, educational, cultural and health care proper, affects the possibilities of promoting, preventing, treating and rehabilitating mental health.

The challenges have been set in the city of Porto Alegre: a growing demand for health activity together with the need to advance in reforming the prevailing health system. The legal foundations have already been established, and it is up to the different levels of government to make more courageous investments and also increase participation of society in matters pertaining to mental health.

Nowadays, the Porto Alegre City is investing 14.62% of the city budget in health care, and US$3 million reforming health services buildings. This means that health care is a priority for the county administration, a significant inversion in the nation context.

For the next years, it is expected that the municipal health care administration will be reinforced, with the consequent increasing of the social control of policies and resources. In doing so, Porto Alegre is anticipating the Brazilian Health System Reform, emphasising the two factors most important to start and maintain the necessary changes.

However, mental health reform is not there merely to provide care to individuals in psychic distress, but also intends to affirm the individual as a citizen, able to interact with and contribute to the social matrix.

REFERENCES

Almeida Filho, N. et al. (1992). Estudo multicêntrico de morbidade psiquiátrica em áreas urbanas brasileiras (Brasília, São Paulo, Porto Alegre). *Revista da Associação Brasileira de Psiquiatria e Associção Psiquiátrica da América Latina 3*, 93–104.

Busnello, E.D. et al. (1992). Morbidade psiquiátrica na população urbana de Porto Alegre. *Jornal Brasileiro de Psiquiatria 10*, 507–512.

Dias, Miriam T.G. (1997). *Os (des)caminhos da política de saúde mental no Rio Grande do Sul: uma* análise da implantação da Lei de Reforma Psiquiátrica. Dissertação de Mestrado em Serviço Social—Pontificia Universidade Católica do Rio Grande do Sul, Porto Alegre.

IBGE. Instituto Brasileiro de Geografia e Estatística (1991). *Censo Demográfico 1991:*

resultados do universo relativos às características da população e dos domicílios. Número 24–Rio Grande do Sul. Rio de Janeiro.

PMPA (Prefeitura Municipal de Porto Alegre) (1996). *Relatório de Indicadores Sociais de Porto* Alegre. Secretaria do Governo Municipal.

PMPA (Prefeitura Municipal de Porto Alegre) (1997). *Porto Alegre e Sua História*. Coordenação de Comunicação Social. Coordenadoria de Relações Públicas.

PNUD. Programa das Nações Unidas para o Desenvolvimento (1996). *Relatório sobre o* Desenvolvimento Humano no Brasil. Rio de Janeiro/IPEA; DF: PNUD.

CHAPTER TEN

Mental health services in Sydney, Australia

Gavin Andrews
Clinical Research Unit for Anxiety Disorders at St Vincent's Hospital and University of New South Wales, Sydney, Australia
Cathy Issakidis
Clinical Research Unit for Anxiety Disorders at St Vincent's Hospital, Sydney, Australia

THE CITY OF SYDNEY, AUSTRALIA

Sydney was founded in 1788 when Captain Phillip arrived from England to establish a penal colony. His fleet landed in Botany Bay, which Captain Cook had described 18 years earlier. Four days later they discovered the jewel that is Sydney Harbour, and located the new settlement there. Sydney was a convict town for 60 years but, despite its brutal beginnings, the city's mixture of pragmatic egalitarianism and plain indifference has transformed it into a thriving multicultural society, that is, wonderfully, a great place to live.

Sydney today: population and characteristics

Sydney, circa 1997, is four million people spread over the area of greater London. Life expectancy for Australians, despite the truncated expectancy among the aboriginal people, is second only to that in Japan. Infant mortality is 570 per 100,000. The population is ageing (0–15 5%, 65 plus 14%), but not as rapidly as in many developed countries, in part because of the effect of waves of migrants from Europe, New Zealand, South America, and now Asia. Seventy percent complete 12 years of schooling, but those with less education find it more difficult to get work. The unemployment rate is 8.5%, but employment patterns are changing, with increasing proportions of the workforce being female and part-time. Eleven percent are identified as living below the poverty line ($440 per week for a family of two adults and two children) and 32% are living on welfare benefits (aged pension 11%, invalid and sickness 3%, sole parent 3%, unemployment 6%).

Sydney for the disadvantaged

At many levels Sydney is a great place for the competent in society to live, but what about those who are disadvantaged? Housing: Home ownership is very high (70%) and no one would choose to rent on a long-term basis. The state government provides subsidised housing for the poor (2.2% of the housing stock) and a small proportion is reserved for the disabled poor, including those with mental disorders. Even so some people are homeless—defined as 'not living in one's own home and do not know where one will be living in two months time'—and the morbidity in this group is considerable, the morbidity being an important risk factor for homelessness rather than the consequence.

Drugs: Smoking marijuana is endemic, (13% have used in the last month) and, as the plant is easily grown, it is difficult to control. Opiates are freely available and can be obtained 'as easily as ordering a pizza' say the newspapers, yet only 2% say they have ever used, and 1% have used in the past month. Cocaine and crack use is not significant. The significant drugs, in terms of health problems, are tobacco and alcohol, but the community is only gradually limiting the use of these legal drugs. They are beginning to realise that illegal drug use will not be eradicated by law enforcement and that strategies of harm minimisation might be more advantageous. 'If I'm a drug addict' patients are reported to reason 'then my hallucinations will stop when I stop doing drugs, whereas if I'm a schizophrenic I'm doomed' (Hannon, 1991). Dual diagnosis treatment strategies for young people are a feature of the better mental health services.

THE ORGANISATION OF HEALTH CARE IN AUSTRALIA

Australia's health system is largely funded by taxation revenue, both from general taxation revenue and from a specific 'Medicare' levy of 1.4% of all taxable income. The Commonwealth Government disburses the majority of these funds to the states and territories to cover the cost of their public hospital and community services. About one-third of the population have private health insurance which offsets the cost of private hospital care, but not of doctors' fees. Mental health services, whether in public hospitals and community clinics, or given by general practitioners and private psychiatrists, are funded in exactly the same way, although the States also maintain a declining stock of stand-alone mental hospitals. In 1994–95 8.5% of the GDP was spent on health, with about one-twentieth of this, nearly two billion dollars, being directed to the recurrent costs of mental health services, public and private, for treatment of mental and substance use disorders.

The National Mental Health Strategy

Until 1992 there was little attempt to coordinate the development of mental health services in each State or Territory but that year the health ministers of the states and territories agreed to adopt a Commonwealth-initiated six year National Mental Health Strategy to reduce the reliance on separate psychiatric hospitals, increase the focus on community-based care, and to mainstream mental health care with other types of health care. This strategy is in its fifth year and considerable progress is being made towards these goals, and towards increasing the funding available. In the first three years the total public sector in-patient beds were reduced by 11% to 40 per 100,000, the reductions being concentrated in the stand-alone hospitals. The in-patient services are mainly general adult (65%), but 27% are designated psychogeriatric, 5% forensic and 3% child and adolescent services. The community mental health workforce in the same time grew to 23 community-based direct care staff per 100,000 population. There are a total of 78 direct care staff per 100,000 in the public sector, so with 23 staff in the community only 35% of the total public sector expenditure is on community services, considerably short of the stated aim of directing half the expenditure into community services to ensure continuity of care.

The National Mental Health Strategy has also implemented a review of legislation to ensure that the relevant mental health acts are appropriate; it has established a National Community Advisory Group with State and Territory branches, but to date only one in three organisations have consumer advisory committees; and it has programmes to ensure that consumers of mental health services have access to housing, community and domiciliary care services, and employment and training opportunities, from which they had been largely excluded.

Private hospitals, the majority being small acute stand-alone psychiatric hospitals, account for 15% of the total in-patient beds, and bring the total number of in-patient beds from 40 to 46 per 100,000. Their patients are less severe and have longer lengths of stay than the patients in the acute public sector units. There are 7.4 FTE private psychiatrists per 100,000. Private psychiatrists see 1.6% of Australians in a year, see most more than once (mean 8, median 3 sessions) a distribution that is skewed by long-term

TABLE 10.1
Recurrent Spending on Mental Health Services, Australia
1994–95

State and territory funded public sector services	61%
Insurance funded private hospital services	7%
Commonwealth funded services and activities:	32%
Private psychiatrists	11%
General Practitioners	8%
Pharmaceutical subsidies	7%
Veterans' services	3%
Mental health strategy	3%
Other	1%
Total (AUD 1.72 billion)	100%

therapy. Private psychiatrists are concentrated in the capital cities and this is a cause for concern.

In summary, Table 10.1 contains the pattern of expenditure on mental health from public and private sources for 1994/95. Australia spends 8.5% of the GDP on health. Mental health services, private and public, account for one-twentieth of this total health budget ($1.72 billion, plus expenditure on drug and alcohol services). Of this 2 billion for mental health, 61% was spent by the States on public sector hospital and community services; and 32% was spent by the Commonwealth on patients seeing private psychiatrists (11%), on people with mental disorders seen by GPs (8%), on subsidies for drugs (7%), and on the mental health strategy (2%). Direct treatment services for substance use disorders are not included in these figures.

Who gets seen by whom

In Tables 10.2 and 10.3 we provide estimates of the number of people likely to meet criteria for a mental disorder, by severity; and the sector of the health service providing for their needs. Clearly there are shortcomings.

Now what does Australia get for 0.425% of the GDP expended on the treatment of patients with mental disorders? A National Survey on Mental Health and Well-Being is being conducted during 1997 and the results are not yet available. However Andrews (1995) presumed that the patterns of morbidity would be similar to those shown in wave 2 of the US Epidemiologic Catchment Area Studies and in the US National Comorbidity Study and sought to relate data on the available workforce in Australia to the demand for services. The estimated prevalence of mental disorders by severity is displayed in Table 10.2. In terms of services delivered, only one-third of the 25% of the population that meet criteria for a mental disorder in any year could, he decided, be receiving treatment from the health services. Of those that are treated, three-quarters will be treated by

TABLE 10.2
Prevalence of Mental Disorders by Severity

Disorder	*Serious Mental Disorder*[a]	*Chronic Mental Disorder*[b]	*Mild or Transient Disorder*[c]	*12 month Total: any Disorder*	*Mental Problem*[d]
Schizophrenia	0.5	0	0	0.5	NK
Any affective disorder	2.1	2.2	5.2	9.5	NK
Any anxiety disorder	1.2	2.2	9.2	12.6	NK
Any substance use disorder[e]	1.0	2.2	6.3	9.5	NK
Total (% of population)	2.9	5.0	18.6	26.5	NK
Total number (Australia)	0.5M	0.9M	3.4M	4.5M	NK

Notes: [a] 'Serious mental disorder' follows the NAMHC guidelines and includes all schizophrenia and related disorders, all bipolar disorder, 20% of major depressive disorder, and 20% of panic disorder and OCD, together with 10% of social phobia (that comorbid with avoidant personality disorder) and 10% of substance use disorder (principally drug dependence). At this level these disorders are chronic and disabling, frequently lead to hospitalisation and require treatment by a specialist mental health or addictive service, or by a very experienced general practitioner.

[b] 'Chronic mental disorders' are present, like the 'serious mental disorders', throughout the 12 month period and are associated with disability (i.e. global assessment of functioning (GAF) ratings of less than 70). They include 25% of all affective disorders, 17% of all anxiety disorders, and 21% of the substance use disorders. Substance dependence is treated by specialist drug and alchol services in all Australian states but general practitioners have an important role to play in treating substance abuse. General practitioners should be competent to manage the other chronic mental disorders.

[c] 'Mild or transient disorder': 70% of all people with mental disorders identified in the health surveys have disorders either so mild as to not handicap or else disorders that remit without treatment within the year. There are many human services outside the funded health system who already attend to such patients (Stress Management Programmes, Counsellors, Psychologists and Clergy; self help groups and programmes such as AA, other non government organisations) but general practitioners and specialist mental health services are often required to see such patients. They should either advise appropriately or refer to the non health system community services.

[d] 'Mental problems': Many persons with mental problems that do not meet citeria for a mental disorder attend psychiatrists and general practitioners. In the Epidemiological Catchment Area study 4.8% of the population sought services from these groups for social or emotional problems but did not meet criteria for disorder. About a third were subthreshold cases of anxiety or depressive disorders and a further third had met criteria for such disorders previously. Both these observations raise the issue as to whether health budgets should be expended in this way. As treatment is effective one would presume that, at least for the third who had once met criteria for a disorder, treatment may be keeping them well. Nevertheless inappropriate use of both inpatient and outpatient facilities was evident for a significant proportion of this 4.8% in the US data and has been demonstrated in Australia although it appears to be less frequent, even if more expensive, when it does occur. Again Doctors should see and refer on or advise that no treatment is necessary.

[e] As persons with one disorder tend to suffer another, the more severe the disorder the greater this possibility, and the totals have been discounted for this comorbidity, by 0.6 in respect to serious mental disorders, by 0.75 in respect to chronic mental disorders, and by 0.9 in respect to mild or transient disorders.

TABLE 10.3
Relation between Individuals with Severe, Chronic, Mild or Transient Mental Disorders; or Mental Problems; and the Number (and %) of Patients in these Categories being Seen by Various Sectors of the Medical Workforce for their Disorders (all Numbers as Thousands)

	Serious Mental Disorder	*Chronic Mental Disorder*	*Mild or Transient Disorder*	*12 month Total: any Disorder*	*Mental Problem*
Total Numbers (000's)	490	850	3162	4500	Not Known
Public mental health service	94 (41%)	33 (6%)	–	127 (9%)	36 (20%)
Private psychiatrists	69 (30%)	92 (17%)	–	161 (12%)	69 (30%)
General practitioners	35 (15%)	402 (72%)	560	997 (74%)	153
Addictive services	30 (13%)	30 (5%)	3	63 (5%)	Not Known
Total patients seen	228	557	563	1348	217
Percent being seen	47%	66%	18%	30%	(100%)

GPs only, one-eighth by private psychiatrists, and one-eighth by public sector mental health services (see Table 10.3).

There was a marked disparity in costs according to the provider of services, with the public sector services costing four times more than the private psychiatrists who in turn were five times more expensive than the GPs. There was evidence that case severity paralleled this cost differential but was not a sufficient explanation. There were no data on outcome to allow evaluation of the effectiveness of treatment in the three sectors. Cost and effectiveness aside, the real problem is that half the people in Australia with serious mental disorders and one-third of the people with chronic and disabling disorders are not being treated by any health service, despite the apparent adequacy, on international benchmarks, of staffing levels, and despite the professional organisation of the services outlined above.

The organisation of mental health services in New South Wales

New South Wales contains six million people, one-third of Australia's population. Fuller Torrey and the US National Alliance for the Mentally Ill are well known for their ratings of services for the seriously mentally ill. Hoult and Burchmore, in conjunction with the consumer group Schizophrenia Australia and the Clinical Research Unit for Anxiety Disorders at this hospital, completed a similar analysis of the Australian public sector services for serious and chronic mental illnesses like schizophrenia. Information was sought by an extensive questionnaire from service providers, administrators, and consumers. They rated New South

Wales as the state with the best overall services: hospital, community, rehabilitation, and housing. The Hoult and Burchmore survey identified the provision of 24–hour community-based services for the seriously mentally ill as the outstanding achievement of the Australian services. Every mental health service in Sydney (population 4 million) has an extended-hours service which can undertake an emergency home assessment 7 days a week. Extended-hours services on such a scale are rare elsewhere in the world. All this would be simple to understand except that New South Wales, the state with the best services at the time, has consistently spent less on mental health per capita than any other state or territory in Australia. The figures in Table 10.4 are for 1994/95 but NSW Department of Health reports for 1995/96 claim that the per capita figure is now at the median value for Australia, $66 per capita, a triumph largely due to finding out where the money actually went, rather than to increased funding.

The Centre for Mental Health in the New South Wales State Government is pursuing an aggressive policy to ensure that the proportion of the state public sector budget allocated to public sector mental health services are spent on those services; that the funds are progressively redistributed until equal amounts are spent on in-patient and non in-patient services (this will mean a continuing reduction in bed numbers to 30 per 100,000,

TABLE 10.4
Excellence of Service for the Seriously Mentally Ill versus Costs and Resources for the six Australian States (1994/5)

	NSW	*VIC*	*SA*	*TAS*	*WA*	*QLD*	*AUS*
Excellence score	21	18	12	10	8	7	
Public sector							
Total expenditure per capita	$49	$72	$66	$67	$63	$50	$58
(Exp on comm services)	($16)	($31)	($22)	($27)	($18)	($13)	($21)
Community staff per 100,000	23	30	28	23	21	16	23
Psychiatric beds per 100,000	40	34	46	53	42	37	34
% beds in general hospitals	41%	22%	25%	33%	42%	37%	34%
Private services							
Expenditure on private psychiatrists per capita	$9	$11	$13	$8	$5	$7	$9
General practitioners per 100,000	118	120	125	124	111	115	118

NSW, New South Wales; VIC, Victoria; SA, South Australia; TAS, Tasmania; WA, Western Australia; QLD, Queensland; AUS, Australia.

perhaps 20 acute beds and 10 longer-stay beds); and that, while 70% of funds will continue to be spent on adult mental health services, the remaining funds should be split between services directed at child and adolescent, and aged persons' mental health services respectively. Clearly the good services provided by New South Wales that were noted in the Hoult and Burchmore report are to be maintained and improved by the new funding strategy which is committed to the implementation of evidenced based medicine and routine outcome measurement.

South Eastern Sydney Area Health Service. The South Eastern Sydney Area Health Service is one of these areas. It is responsible for providing public sector health care to 727,000 people spread across 300 square kilometres. The area consists of hectare after hectare of detached dwellings of typical Australians—17% of non-English speaking background, 13% over 64 years, 17% under 15, 7.5% unemployed, 37% with private health insurance. This Area Health Service receives $43 per capita to support the public sector health services, significantly less that the state average of $52. The South Eastern Sydney Area Health Service mental health services are deployed in four sectors. This report will focus on the northern sector in which St. Vincent's Hospital provides services to the permanent and transient inhabitants of the inner city, an area that now comprises both the central business district and the centre for sleaze. It wasn't always so.

ST. VINCENT'S HOSPITAL SERVICES FOR THE INNER CITY SECTOR

In 1863, medical opinion was outraged that lunatics were admitted to gaol prior to being transferred to an asylum and called for the establishment of a 'Lunatic Receiving House' where people could be assessed in humane surroundings and treatment started promptly. A pleasant building was erected and the first patients were admitted in 1868. Located adjacent to the police station and the court house, and across the street from the gaol, the Reception House functioned for 93 years as the only centre in the state for the triage of the mentally ill. By 1961, when it was closed, it was admitting people at the rate of 10 per day into what had become a 30 bed facility that concentrated on the prompt assessment and transfer of patients to a mental hospital, to a private hospital, or back into the community. By then, the emphasis on treatment in mental hospitals was diminishing and the emphasis on treatment in general hospital units with associated community services had begun. In 1961 the building was renovated and extended and reopened under the aegis of the Sisters of Charity as the Caritas Centre, a 36 bed psychiatric unit, part of St.

Vincent's Hospital, a teaching hospital of the University of New South Wales.

In 1986 the Clinical Research Unit for Anxiety Disorders was established as a joint endeavour between the university and the hospital. In 1988 the small community health centre in the area was significantly enlarged and located in the old police station next door, the jail across the road having become a technical college some 70 years earlier. The community and hospital services are in the process of being formally integrated even though they have worked as one service since the community clinic was relocated in 1988. In 1994 a liaison service to the general hospital was established and in 1996 a liaison service for local GPs was established. This conglomerate of services, the St. Vincent's Mental Health Services, has all the usual paraphernalia of conglomerates—directors, deputy directors, business managers, research units, medical informatics units, catering units—likely to be of benefit to patients.

Specifically, the tasks that the Service undertakes—and in part, they are the tasks that any mental health service should undertake—are, circa 1997, listed below and then discussed in turn.

1. Provide a hospital and community service to meet the needs of the local population.
2. Provide a super speciality service to meet the need for centres of excellence in the common mental disorders, namely the anxiety disorders.
3. Provide a liaison service to meet the needs of the general hospital patients.
4. Provide a liaison service to meet the needs of the local GPs.
5. Provide an educational programme to support these initiatives.
6. Provide a consumer liaison programme so that the services continue to meet the articulated needs of consumers and voluntary agencies.
7. Conduct research and evaluation on the quality of health outcomes.

The hospital and community service to meet the needs of the local population

The local catchment area is small, some 72,000 population although, when weighted for known risk factors it rises to the equivalent of 186,000 ordinary Australians. The demography of the area is that of most inner areas in large cities. While few people, apart from the wealthy in high rise apartment blocks, live in the central business district, the immediate surrounding area is densely populated. The old low rise buildings are a rabbit warren of shops, homes, small businesses, apartments, hotels, rooming houses, shelters for the homeless and premises used for prostitution and drugs. The contrast between the neat and tidy central business district and the sleaze to the east is marked. While the age standardised mortality ratios in the whole South Eastern Area Health Service are lower than the Australian norms, those in the inner city catchment area are higher, and the excess mortality is due to drugs, AIDS, alcoholic hepatitis, and suicide, which probably describe the local population better than the following, dry population statistics. Compared to the rest of New South Wales the people in the area are less likely to be born in Australia (47% *vs* 75%), less likely to be living in the same residence as five years ago (34% *vs* 56%), more likely to be renting (57% *vs* 25%) and more likely to be living in single person households (46% *vs* 7%). There are fewer than expected children and aged.

The Inner City Mental Health Service (Budget: $5,450,000)

Aims. The stated aims are legion and impractical. In practice the service is very clear that it exists to serve the needs of the region; responding to crises, offering short-term hospitalisation and long-term case management in the community, and doing whatever is necessary to maintain the deprived and damaged clientele as untroubled by their psychoses as possible. It is not, and can not be, a resource for all whose mental state leads them to behave badly, no matter how desperately some would wish it to be so. Health services are rationed and this service is clear about the priorities.

Structure. The physical structure was constructed in 1967 for voluntary patients and was not designed for the current clientele. The 27 bed in-patient unit is equivalent to 37.5 beds per 100,000, just under the present state average and probably appropriate given the high levels of morbidity in the area (equivalent to 15 beds per 100,000 weighted population, but there is no access to the 10 longer-stay beds envisaged in the planning documents). The in-patient unit was constructed on land adjacent to the 1867 'Lunatic Reception House' which is now used as offices. The community mental health centre is housed in the adjacent 1867 police station, though the police cells which survive are used for storage and not for people. This mental health facility of community clinic and in-patient unit is separated from the main hospital by a small urban park and by the old jail, about 400m, although it seems much further on a dark night. The service has 22 cars and sufficient mobile telephones to enable it to be a proactive outreach service.

Staffing. The Inner City Mental Health Service has 100 staff, 55% are trained psychiatric nurses, 18% are occupational therapists, social workers or psychologists, 10% are psychiatrists and trainee psychiatrists, and the remaining 17% are non-clinical support staff. Many staff work on both the community and in-patient services but the community mental health centre has the full time equivalent of 50 clinical staff for a population of 72,000, three times the state and national averages, but on target at 20 per 100,000 weighted average, given the morbidity in the area. The in-patient unit is staffed at the state average for acute units, 1.2 clinical staff per bed. The aim of NSW Department of Health is to have budget expenditure equally divided between in-patient and community services. This is one service in which the budget is evenly divided.

Function. The in-patient unit functions like any acute in-patient unit, or at least like any in-patient unit that services an inner city clientele. A census of a 1995 cohort of admissions showed that 52% had psychosis, mostly recurrent, that 10% were from out of the area and had gravitated to the area after becoming ill, that 16% were of no fixed abode, that 33% were admitted as involuntary patients under the various provisions of the state mental health act, and that 40% were brought by the police as being an acute danger to themselves or others. Using the Health of the Nation Outcome Scale, the staff rated the patients as very severe on admission, but considered that they had made one standard deviation improvement before discharge to community care an average of 10 days later. Compared to other units in the study, this unit was the most efficient in terms of improvement per day of stay, a creditable achievement given such a severe and deprived clientele. To what can we attribute this achievement? First there was a close liaison with the community mental health teams, second there was a high level of professionalism among the staff many of whom had worked in the system long enough to know many patients well, and third that each patient was presented to all staff on a daily basis so that clinical decision making was informed and prompt. Last, the unit has a strong focus on educating each patient about their illness and the rationale for their treatment.

Community mental health centre. The community mental health centre is clever, and this originality has resulted in a number of awards for excellence. It was comprehensively evaluated in 1990–95 (Teesson, 1996). It functions in three teams with distinct roles, though of course there is a considerable overlap in what staff in each team actually do. The Crisis team responds to calls for help from police, medical practitioners, voluntary agencies, and the general population. Always available, the crisis team can see people at the community mental health centre, at home or at the site of the crisis immediately, 24 hours a day, 7 days per week. If the person is known to the service or there is another health professional in attendance then one staff member can go, if the crisis is acute and emergency diagnosis and treatment may be indicated then two or three staff can attend, including the registrar. The Crisis team also services the hostels for the homeless in the area and, supported by Honorary Medical Staff, has, for a number of years, conducted evening clinics in the major shelters, assessing patients and prescribing the relevant medication. An elegant time series analysis (Buhrich & Teesson, 1996) showed that these clinics had, after a period of increased case ascertainment, enabled people with psychosis, who would otherwise have been treated in hospital, to be treated in the community, even though they had no fixed abode. Teesson also showed that consumers and shelter bed staff were satisfied with the response of the Crisis team.

The Case Management team follows the clinical case manager model not the brokerage model. The team is represented at the morning reviews on the ward and ensures that every patient resident in the area is assessed for suitability for case management prior to discharge. The team members take clinical responsibility for the day to day management of all patients (one day census, total case load = 630) liaising with the consultant as necessary. In a triumph of scheduling, every active case is reviewed by all members of the team at least every six months and, if necessary, a new management plan effected. Teesson (1996) followed 93 chronically homeless people with psychosis for one year and showed that while they are of no fixed abode they do tend to remain in the same geographic area. They are therefore appropriate for long-term case management, even if finding them on any particular day might be problematic. This is where experienced case managers who know the area do so well.

The third, or extended care and rehabilitation team, takes responsibility for the most severely ill patients and, in the shortage of long-stay supervised accommodation, manages them with a combination of intensive case management and attendance at a living skills and rehabilitation centre. Teesson and Hambridge (1992) showed that intensive case management was a cost effective option in general, and it was cost neutral even for such a disabled and deprived group as seen by the Rehabilitation team. Teesson (1996) also delineated the level of disability and the very slow response to rehabilitation in this group, and one might ask whether some of these patients might benefit from an intensive period of in-patient rehabilitation were such facilities available. Either way it is clear that the rehabilitation team is inhibiting deterioration and minimising harm from the violence and drugs which are prevalent in this part of the city.

The crisis team sees people in crisis, the case management team deals with those needing continued treatment and the rehabilitation team is concerned with people with end stage psychosis. The Inner City Mental Health Service has other initiatives which support these core activities. A small group are actively involved with young people with early psychosis and seek, by caring about engagement, optimal treatment of psychosis, family intervention and maintenance of education or employment, to effectively alter the course of the illness. This is a new initiative and no results are available. One staff member is concerned with aboriginal patients and, as such, is unusual in Sydney, despite the considerable morbidity and mortality in this population. Another staff member liaises with the non-government organisations that provide the bulk of the accommodation in the community for people disabled by serious mental illness, with the local consumer groups, and with government agencies. The service has also found it necessary to have formal agreements with the police, and with the accident and emergency department of the hospital. Outcome is not yet measured as a routine even though it has proved quite practical to do so in specific studies on the ward and in the community clinic.

The Clinical Research Unit for Anxiety Disorders

In 1985 St. Vincent's Hospital, realising that the Department of Psychiatry was almost totally focused on the seriously mentally ill, took advantage of the offer of a small anxiety disorders unit's wish to relocate from another hospital, if only because that unit might broaden the reputation and educational experience available at the hospital. The psychoses are relatively rare diseases that commonly disable and when severe cause public affront and make it imperative that something be done. In the burden of disease studies schizophrenia and bipolar affective disorder account for 3.5% of the burden of human disease in developed countries like Australia. In contrast the anxiety disorders are common disorders, but because they are less likely to disable, and because the sufferers go to great pains not to cause affront to family or friends, the need for treatment appears minimal. Yet the burden of disease studies, which did not include the phobias, still found that the anxiety disorders contributed more to the burden of human disease (2.2%) than either bipolar affective disorder or schizophrenia. An anxiety disorders clinic and a mood disorders clinic should be part of every comprehensive psychiatric service if the aim of that service is to treat people disabled by mental disorders and not simply to deal with medico-social emergencies. The New South Wales Department of Health has accepted, but not yet specifically funded, Centres of Excellence in the significant mental disorders. The Clinical Research Unit for Anxiety Disorders has been so nominated.

The Clinical Research Unit for Anxiety Disorders (Budget: $244,000 clinic; $240,000 research (external funds)

Structure and function. The Anxiety Disorders Clinic occupies the cottage built for the Superintendent of the Lunatic Reception House at the turn of the century. Situated between the old Reception House building and the old police station it makes an excellent clinic. The clinic has a full time equivalent staff of five and specialises in cognitive behaviour therapy for people with anxiety disorders (Andrews, 1996), and these treatment programmes have been published (Andrews, Crino, Hunt, Lampe, & Page, 1994). Only referred patients are seen. The clinic is a tertiary referral service and does not see people in crisis and does not offer stress management or long-term counselling. It gives preference to people referred by psychiatrists and clinical psychologists. Seven hundred new patients, two-thirds from outside the South Eastern Sydney Area Health Service catchment area, are seen each year and about half are accepted for treatment. The remainder are referred back to their doctor with advice about the appropriate diagnosis (usually depression presenting as an anxiety disorder) and treatment. Once people are offered treatment, of 20 to 80 hours duration, depending on diagnosis, most accept and 83% complete. Drop outs are very rare, a tribute to the excellence of the treatment. Outcome assessment, in part computerised, is a routine and the results are published.

The Clinical Research Unit for Anxiety Disorders was developed on the idea that if one had basic researchers at one end of the corridor and clinicians at the other, and they all took tea together, then both would be informed. The model for this was the Burden Neurological Institute in Bristol that, 25 years earlier, had had artificial intelligence people and neurologists occupy the same tea room in the hope that they would talk. To some extent this cross fertilisation has happened in Sydney, increasingly the clinicians are doing their own basic research and the six researchers, now funded by external grants, are active in other fields. The Unit has been made a World Health Organization Collaborating Centre in Mental Health and Substance Abuse with special responsibility for diagnostic interviews and treatment protocols. As such it plays a central role in the WHO Composite International Diagnostic Interview; being responsible for the anxiety disorders modules, for the data entry programme and scorer for the whole interview, and for the CIDI-Auto, a computerised version of the interview. It is currently funded to examine the validity of the psychosis module of the CIDI and, if possible, improve it. The unit has been active in the assessment of outcome measures and has developed the interview for the current Australian National Survey of Mental Health and Well-Being. The epidemiological analysis of these data will inform the debate about the appropriate weightings for mental disorders in the burden of disease studies (Andrews & Sanderson, 1997) and for disentangling the burden in comorbid conditions. In terms of treatment protocols it completed the series on Treatment Outlines for Australian psychiatrists in 1991 (Quality Assurance Project, 1991), contributed to the World Health Organization initiatives in this area, has published a widely used text on the management of mental disorders (Treatment Protocol Project, 1997), and is preparing a text on the management of acute in-patient units in psychiatry. Maybe taking tea with the clinicians was successful after all.

The liaison service to meet the needs of the general hospital patients

The Division of Mental Health Services has always been pleased to offer a consultation service to the general hospital. It was simply part of the camaraderie of medicine. The haematologist or registrar came to see your patient and you or your registrar went to see their patient. Occasionally more time would be spent when the apparent needs of the general hospital fitted with the interests of one of the psychiatrists. In early years these special interests included the pain clinic and more latterly the neuropsychological manifestations of HIV/AIDS. In 1990, the College of Psychiatrists altered its training requirements to make a term in liaison psychiatry essential. It was time for firm action, especially as St. Vincent's was host to groundbreaking initiatives in heart and bone marrow transplantation, and in HIV/AIDS, all of which expressed the need for liaison psychiatric help.

The General Hospital Liaison Service (Budget: $330,000)

Structure and function. In 1994 a liaison psychiatrist was appointed, supported by a registrar on a training rotation, and two part-time senior nurses. In 1996 a formal liaison psychiatry unit was established, located within the general hospital, and latterly supported by a specialist psychiatrist (part-time), and a clinical psychologist. The current ethos is to emphasise early detection and the education of other clinicians to manage liaison cases themselves. However, in addition to the units mentioned above, Liaison now services the Accident and Emergency Service, seeing as a priority, people held overnight for psychiatric opinion. They also play a planned role in oncology, as well as responding to consultation requests from all hospital units.

The liaison service to meet the needs of the local general practitioners

Three-quarters of the people in Australia who do meet criteria for a mental disorder and who see a doctor see a GP who diagnoses and treats without specialist advice. General practitioners find it difficult to form a consulting relationship with psychiatrists like they do with most other specialists, simply because psychiatrists are loath to take their phone calls. The federal government commissioned an inquiry which recommended a change in the payment structure for private psychiatrists so that they were rewarded more for consulting and less for continued psychotherapy. In another initiative, the government made money available for shared care programmes in which psychiatrists would meet regularly with GPs to discuss the management of general practice cases. The St. Vincent's Hospital Psychiatric Service, overwhelmed by the demands of the indigent psychotic patient has, until recently, stood back from any liaison with GPs.

A liaison service for general practitioners (Budget: $220,000)

Structure and function. In 1996 a senior psychiatrist experienced in affective disorders and in shared care consultations with GPs was appointed to develop a general practitioner liaison programme. The first steps have involved a continuation of the shared care consultations, now in respect to GPs in the catchment area; an exploration by videotape of GPs competencies in interviewing an actor simulating depression, and planned interventions with consultation and instructional materials to assist GPs in the recognition and management of bipolar affective disorder.

The educational programme to support these initiatives

The whole service is part of St. Vincent's Hospital, a teaching hospital of the University of New South Wales. A programme of clinical training for fifth year medical students is undertaken and, at any time, nine students are doing placements in the various sections of the service. Clinical placements are also offered to students of nursing and clinical psychology. The Clinical Research Unit for Anxiety Disorders has long felt that there is little point in excellence unless you teach others. For 10 years they have taught medical students and trainee psychiatrists about the anxiety disorders, they have conducted workshops on issues of the day, such as Falloon's ideas about the management of the seriously mentally ill, and they have offered placements and courses to people wanting to learn what the unit does, whether that be the treatment of anxiety disorders, the use of the CIDI and the Personality Disorder Examination, or the measurement of outcome. For six years they have offered, as a University of NSW Masters programme, a two year part time course in psychological medicine for general practitioners. This masters programme, which next year will be able to be taken by distance education over the internet, aims to teach experienced GPs how to recognise and treat patients with mental disorders who present within their own practices. The Management of Mental Disorders (see p. 206) is widely used by GPs throughout Australia.

Educational programmes: St. Vincent Hospital Certificate Courses (Budget: $45,000)

In 1996 an education officer was appointed to organise a more comprehensive series of St. Vincent's Hospital Certificate Courses. The first courses were for psychiatrists and clinical psychologists in cognitive behaviour therapy and in recent advances in therapeutics; for nurses new to community mental health nursing in strategies of value in the community; and for all clinicians in topics as diverse as research methods, management of people with personality disorders, or the organisation of mental health services. In all, 2400 person days are being offered to health professionals from all over New South Wales.

The consumer liaison programme

Australian mental health services were relatively unconcerned with the views of consumers or carers until they developed a political presence in the late 1980s. The National Enquiry into the Human Rights of People with Mental Illness was, if anything, the turning point. There are now many strong advocate groups in mental health, both at the state and national level. The Commonwealth has established a National Consumer Advisory Group which has state branches and which takes input from the various organisations. To some extent these organisations reflect the traditional groupings and while there are advocates for schizophrenia and for bipolar disorder there are no advocates for unipolar major depression, the disorder of greatest burden. There were no advocates for anxiety disorders either until a group in South Australia founded the Anxiety Disorder Foundation of Australia. The anxiety disorders clinic at St. Vincent's Hospital was pleased to assist in the founding of a New South Wales branch which now is independent and has more than 800 members. There is a serious need for a similar body to represent people with depression.

Consumer representatives are now required for most federally funded programmes, to the extent that most consumers who are at all active are being worn out by their commitments. The Inner City Mental Health Service has consumers on the two patient care committees which meet monthly. Consumers also attend the senior staff meeting. The Anxiety Disorder Clinic has a bill of patient rights and, by distributing copies of each treatment programme at the beginning of treatment, ensures that each patient knows what to expect and can complain if certain elements of treatment are not made available. All patients are debriefed at the end of treatment, the responses recorded and identified problems rectified.

Evaluating the quality of health outcomes

All sensible services should spend a fixed proportion of their budgets on research and development. To some extent teaching hospitals, in exchange for the cost of teaching students, have gained from the research ideas of the academics. But proper R&D is more than academic interest in new developments, it is about quality assurance that services are being run properly, and that health gains are being achieved.

Research and Evaluation Unit (Budget: $45,000)

When the Community Health Centre was established in 1988 a research officer was appointed whose tasks were overseen by a triumvirate of two senior service personnel and an academic. Their task was to ensure that the research officer did not simply deliquesce into the CEO's personal assistant, into someone who only gathered data to answer the pressing questions of the day. Given such protection, the incumbent produced a body of quality assurance research (Teesson, 1996) that was fed back to, and influenced, the functioning of the Service. Donabedian would have been proud.

REFLECTIONS: PAST AND FUTURE

The Inner City Mental Health Service has adequate staff and facilities to provide a comprehensive psychiatric service to the people of the inner city. It does this well. The service is multidisciplinary and sensitive to consumer feedback. The service is a proactive outreach service that can provide a 24 hours a day service throughout the sector. One marker of success is that Sydney, unlike many other large cities, does not have numbers of apparently psychotic individuals shambling about. Sydney should be, and to a large extent is, grateful to the St. Vincent's Mental Health Service. What then are the problems? The principal problem is the rising tide of gratuitous violence among those being treated. Some of this is explained by the increase in the use of illegal drugs, especially amphetamines and steroids. But some is due to a change in societal perceptions of respect due to health professionals. There is an increasing shortage of nurses, doctors and other health professionals who want to work in public sector psychiatry and especially who want to treat those who are chronically psychotic. Unfortunately, there is little evidence that treatment of chronic psychosis materially alters the long-term prognosis of the disorder and this, coupled with a difficult and dangerous work environment, makes recruiting good staff for New South Wales public sector acute services very difficult. To date staffing levels in the Inner City Service have been able to be maintained because of this unit's reputation for excellence, and because the mission statement of the Sisters of Charity encourages like-minded staff to serve. But fame and altruism are poor grounds for long-term planning and this problem of the working environment will have to be solved.

The demand for the treatment programmes offered by the Anxiety Disorders Clinic is overwhelming. About four times as many patients are referred as can be seen and treated. Even if there was money we would be reluctant to expand. Thus we tend to see only people who are suitable for and who desire treatment with cognitive behaviour therapy. Success has been a straitjacket and to some extent has narrowed the field of interest so that the Clinic is not as broadly based as a centre of excellence should be. As a consequence we are deliberately branching out into the management of hypochondriasis, and other stress, anxiety and somatoform disorders.

While the desire of psychiatrists to be seen as part of medicine is understandable, the cost offset of providing a liaison service has never been completely clear. The existence of a liaison service often excuses physicians and surgeons from practising whole person medicine with difficult patients—'get the liaison fellow to fix it' is the cry. We have often wondered whether an educational programme for physicians and surgeons might be more cost-effective, and it remains to be seen whether the current emphasis on clinician education will prove fruitful. Nevertheless, the existence of liaison psychiatry encourages general hospital services to see psychiatry as the place for difficult people, a sort of oubliette for the patient nobody else wants. Given that the acute in-patient unit has a mean stay of 10 days, a charter to deal with acute and serious mental disorders, and is replete with many wild and dangerous people, this hope is seriously wrong. It is important that private and public sector psychiatrists be seen as one specialist mental health resource and many private psychiatrists do continue to support the public sector. Public sector services however have been loath to support private psychiatrists.

It is far too early to pass comment on the general practitioner liaison service, but unless the rift between GPs and psychiatry is also bridged, we will see ill-informed treatment for half the people who meet criteria for a mental disorder and that, circa 1997, is simply untenable. More importantly, unipolar major depression was identified as the leading cause of disability, world wide, in 1990 (Murray & Lopez, 1996). New data on the poor outcome to be expected from the routine treatment of depressive illness (Andrews, Neilson, Hunt, Stewart, & Kiloh, 1990) makes it clear that GPs who see the vast majority of cases will have to become very sophisticated in the management of this disorder if the level of disablement due to this treatable disorder is to be lessened. If burden of disease is any guide then we should be putting twice as much money into the treatment of unipolar major depression than to the treatment of schizophrenia. At present this service spends an order of magnitude less, but is better than most. At least it realises the problem.

The education programmes are a success story. People from outside St. Vincent's seem eager to pay to attend and one would hope that these people would decide that St. Vincent's is an exciting place to work and so apply when vacancies are advertised. Informed and articulate consumers are overworked and, while governments see that the appointment of a consumer representative to a project or treatment centre might absolve them of blame if something goes wrong, it is simply too much to expect of the available consumers at this point. There is another concern. The purpose of medicine is to get people well so that they never have to see a doctor again. Identification with a consumer group can maintain the sick or damaged role, whereas the person might be better off being identified as healthy. All disorders benefit from pressure groups, after all the traditional method of funding is the same as last year plus or minus 5% for pressure groups. The problem is that not all people benefit from working for such pressure groups. Sometimes working for a pressure group is not the best way for a recovered patient to spend the rest of their life. Or for a grieving parent. The service is presently under considerable pressure to do more with less. Predictably the research officer is being consumed by the need to support the director. In the short term this is understandable, but in the longer term the service will benefit from an independent research initiative that seeks to develop programmes to inform the service rather than simply answer current questions.

The WHO/World Bank project on the Burden of Disease may offer a way to combine equity and efficiency. They report (Murray & Lopez, 1996) that in established market economies, 22% of the total burden of human disease, measured in disability adjusted life years lost, is due to mental and substance use disorders. Furthermore they have argued (Bobadilla, Cowley, Musgrove, & Saxenian, 1994), that as no country can afford to meet the needs of the total population one should apportion health services according to the burden of a disease and the cost-effectiveness of dealing with it. Mental and substance use disorders account for 22% of the burden, but in Australia only get 5–6% of the total health budget. Clearly a substantial increase in funding is in order, even before we go into the cost-effectiveness of treatment.

If there was such a budget windfall, we should apportion it to the various mental disorders in proportion to their burden (affective disorders 8.5%, substance use disorders 6.3%, dementia 2.9%, anxiety disorders 2.4% and schizophrenia 2.3%). At present the St. Vincent's Mental Health Services apportion at least 50% to psychosis and at most 20% to the depressive and anxiety disorders in total. Even so, this service is leading the way in terms of distributing resources according to burden. Nevertheless, one would hope to be able to progressively apportion funds according to probability of health gain, and not according to society's need to respond to demand or to limit the affront that people with psychotic disorders can cause. We think that carers share this concern, even if the affront is as hard to bear as the sickness. The burden of disease figures are first approximations and will surely change. Judging from our pilot data, the total burden of disease due to mental disorders will stay stable, while the relative importance but not the rank order of the disorders will change. That is, the largest burden will be due to the affective disorders and the most cost-effective treatments will be those associated with the anxiety disorders. In burden and cost-effectiveness terms therefore, more money should be spent on the depressive and anxiety disorders if the country wishes to be productive and rich. People who can be cured, but who remain disabled at home, are an affront to our humanity as well as being an avoidable drain on the economic well being of all. Which accords with our view of the purpose of specialist medicine, which is to heal people and never need to see them again.

REFERENCES

Andrews, G. (1995). Workforce deployment: reconciling demands and resources. *Australian and New Zealand Journal of Psychiatry, 29*, 394–402.

Andrews, G. (1996), Talking therapies that work: the rise of cognitive behaviour therapy. Editorial. *British Medical Journal, 313*, 1501–1502.

Andrews, G., Neilson, M., Hunt, C., Stewart, G., & Kiloh, L.G. (1990). Diagnosis, personality and the long-term outcome of depression. *British Journal of Psychiatry, 157*, 13–18.

Andrews, G., Crino, R., Hunt, C., Lampe, L., & Page, A. (1994). *The treatment of anxiety disorders.* New York: Cambridge University Press.

Andrews, G. & Sanderson, K. (1997). The burden of disease in panic disorder and obsessive compulsive disorder. In C.J.L. Murray and A.D. Lopez (Eds) *The global burden of disease and injury series. VI Neuro-psychiatric disorders.* Boston: Harvard School of Public Health.

Bobadilla, J.-L., Cowley, P., Musgrove, P., & Saxenian, H. (1994). Design, content and financing of an essential national package of health services. In C.J.L. Murray and A.D. Lopez (Eds) *Global comparative assessments in the health sector,* (pp. 171–180). Geneva: World Health Organisation.

Buhrich, N. & Teesson, M. (1996). Impact of a psychiatric outreach service for homeless persons with schizophrenia. *Psychiatric Services, 47*, 644–646.

Hannon, L. (1991). *Stigma, felt identity and the chronic mentally ill.* Unpublished PhD Thesis, Department of Anthropology, University of Sydney, Sydney.

Murray, C.J.L. & Lopez, A.D. (Eds) (1996). *The global burden of disease.* Boston: Harvard University Press.

Quality Assurance Project, The (1991). Treatment outlines for antisocial personality disorder. *Australian and New Zealand Journal of Psychiatry, 25*, 541–547.

Teesson, M. (1996). *An evaluation of mental health service delivery in an inner city area.* Unpublished PhD thesis, University of New South Wales, Sydney.

Teesson, M. & Hambridge, J. (1992). Mobile community treatment in inner city and suburban Sydney. *Psychiatric Quarterly, 63*, 119–127

Treatment Protocol Project (1997). *Management of Mental Disorders, 2nd Edition.* World Health Organisation Collaborating Centre for Mental Health and Substance Abuse: Darlinghurst NSW.

CHAPTER ELEVEN

Mental health in Tehran in the context of the national mental health programme of Iran

Ahmad Mohit
Iran University of Medical Science, Iran

GENERAL FACTS ABOUT IRAN

Iran is a vast country covering about 1,600,000 km^2 located in south-western Asia. Over half of the area is covered by mountains, a quarter is desert, and less than one-quarter arable land. This variety in the environment has entailed dramatic variations in the socio-economic and cultural state of the people, from the prosperous, fertile green fields and forests of the humid north, to the dry, unfriendly desert sands of the centre.

According to the last national census of 1996, the population of the country is 60 million of which 60.4% live in urban and 39.6% in rural areas. The average size of the family is just less than five persons. The Iranian family of today can best be described as a family in transition from extended structure to nuclear arrangement, therefore prone to many stresses. The population is quite young and the average age is just less than 20 years. Recent efforts at population control have been quite successful, and the annual population increase has dropped from over 3.5 in 1986 to 1.4 in 1996. The overall literacy rate is 80%, representing 85% of the population in urban and 74% in rural areas. The literacy rate among women is close to 70%. Ninety-six percent of children reaching school age, enroll in schools, making the total number of students in the current scholastic year 20 million. There are also close to 1 million university students. Until recently, the country's economy has been oil-dependent, but during the last decade, both agricultural and industrial sectors have been gaining a share in the overall economy. The official language and script is Persian. About 99% of the people are Muslims (91% Shiite and 8.5% Sunni), 0.2% are Christian, 0.07% Zoroastrian and 0.05% Jewish. Since the 1979 revolution the country's political system has changed from a kingdom to an Islamic Republic.

Iran is divided into 28 administrative provinces (*Ostan*). Each province is divided into a number of districts (*Shahrestan*) of which the country has about 250, more than 500 cities (*Shahr*), 600 sub-districts or towns (*Bakhsh*) and over 66,000 villages (*Roostaa*). The capital city of Iran, Tehran, is also the centre of a province with the same name. More than 10 million out of 36 million urban Iranians live in the Greater Tehran Area, therefore making it a major urban centre, or a so called *mega city.*

The city of Tehran

Natural location and history. The capital city of Iran, Tehran is situated on the southern slopes of the Alborz mountains that separate the Caspian sea from mainland Iran. The city lies at an average altitude of 1100 m above the sea level and is the largest and the most populous city in Iran. Tehran, which means 'warm slope', was a village in the suburb of the ancient Iranian capital of 'Rey'. Following the fall of 'Rey' to Mongols in 1220 AD, the residents of this city moved to Tehran and the foundation for this small village to become a city was thus laid. The visitor of today's Tehran, can hardly believe the 9th century account of a historian of the same city: 'Tehran is one of the villages of Rey with such untamed inhabitants, who are not only insurgent against their governors, but are in constant clashes among themselves to the extent that travelling between its twelve quarters has become impossible and they are inevitably forced to build and live in underground dwellings resembling ant nests'. The real growth and gradual distinction of Tehran started in the 16th century and reached its culmination in the late 18th century when it was chosen by the founder of Qajaar dynasty to be the capital city of Iran.

During the late 19th and early 20th centuries, Tehran was the centre of dramatic developments of constitutional revolution that was the beginning of a long, and at times painful road, of constructing modern Iran. With the fall of the Qajaar dynasty, a western model of restructuring became the order of the day. It was in this city that Iran's first modern university and hospitals were built. Tehran became a famous capital during the Second World War, where Churchill, Roosevelt and Stalin had one of their most famous meetings. Once more it became famous during the movement for nationalisation of oil in early 1950s. Finally it gained its highest fame in 1978 when it became the centre of most important activities and demonstrations of the Islamic revolution. After the revolution and for the most part of the decade of 1980s, Iran was involved in a war with neighbouring Iraq. The war had devastating effects on many parts of the country including Tehran, that was a target of bombings and missile attacks and also a destination for many refugees. In addition, there were the problems of neighbouring Afghanistan and the flow of refugees from that country. Such conditions caused many disruptions in the life of the city. Therefore, it would not be an exaggeration if we talk of the years 1980–1987 as the worst years of modern Tehran.

The war ended in 1988 and soon after, the programmes for reconstruction of the country started. During the eight years of reconstruction, Tehran has gone through tremendous change. On the one hand the city is visibly cleaner. Large areas of green space have been created and an extensive highway system has eased the traffic. The construction of an underground railway is almost finished without foreign financial or essential technical assistance. Finally, a number of cultural centres and libraries have been built in all parts of the city, particularly poor neighbourhoods of south Tehran. On the other hand, these developments have been accompanied by a dramatic change in lifestyle. Gradually, living in high rises is becoming the norm. There are new and huge construction sites visible everywhere. Many of these new dwellings are occupied by first or second generation young couples who have come to Tehran in search of a better income and a brighter future. Old, solemn houses with peaceful courtyards and gatherings of extended family members, are, for the most part, things of the past. Only the privileged few, or an odd old couple living in a rare, intact corner of a traditional neighbourhood can afford such luxuries. Tehran is thus in transition. Both as a city and population-wise it is relatively young. It does not enjoy the same charm, and rich heritage of history and culture of a city like Cairo or Isfahan. Tehran's main resource is dynamism of youth and a willingness to create an identity. With this come many stresses, and to face them there have been innovations.

Demography. According to the most recent national census of 1996, the population of Tehran is about 7 million. However, considering many suburban areas and settlements around the city, it is safe to say that at least about 10 million people depend on this city every day. According to the first official census of Tehran, taken in 1883, the population of this city was 106,482. In 1922 the city's inhabitants were 210,000. In 1939 this number was increased to 540,000. Tehran's population shows a threefold increase from 1,512,000 in 1956 to 4,530,000 in 1976. The population of the city in 1986 was just above 6 million. The population of Tehran is quite young and the ratio of the age group 0–20 years of age is more than 40%.

In general, Tehran's affluent neighbourhoods are in the northern part of the city, and as one goes towards the south, inhabitants become more deprived. This is reflected in per-capita income, housing space, public facilities, educational and health facilities, and the like.

Like all other major cities, provision of health care in Tehran is through a complex combination of public, private, insurance, and special services, such as the ones for military personnel and their families. Distribution of these services is not even. Most of the population of poor and condensed areas is unable to use private services, and poorer neighbourhoods depend for most of their needs on governmental services that are overcrowded and strained.

THE HEALTH SYSTEM

Iran is a signatory to the World Health Organisation (WHO) sponsored Alma-Ata declaration of 1978, aiming at Health for All by the Year 2000. Moving in this direction during the past two decades, the country's health system and indicators have been improving steadily. This has been achieved through a network of primary health care systems in rural and urban areas and is being coordinated at the national level by the Ministry of Health and Medical Education. This ministry is responsible for all aspects of planning, leadership, supervision and evaluation of health services in the country, including training of human resources for health at all levels. In 1996, the Iranian Ministry of Health and Medical Education received 6.7% of the national budget, 4.2% of the GNP, of which 37% was devoted to local health services. The per capita annual budget of the Ministry of Health and Medical Education has been US$92.

Provincial level

At the provincial level, there are 32 Universities of Medical Sciences and Health Services. In addition to all scientific functions and responsibilities of a university, they are in charge of all the health needs of a certain geographic area of the country. They function independently under the general rules and policies set by the Ministry. In each province the health affairs are run by one of these universities. Only Tehran province is divided among three major universities. The executive authority of the chancellor of the university is exercised through his different deputies, including the deputy for health affairs.

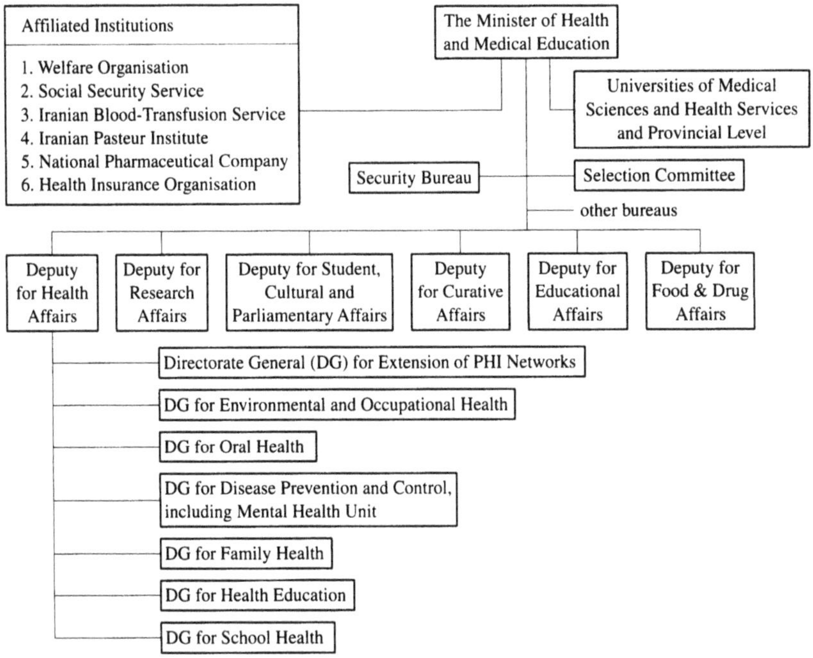

FIG. 11.1 A brief organisational chart of the Iranian health system is shown above.

District level

Each one of such universities oversees the activities of the next level; that is, the district level. The district is the smallest autonomous unit in Iran's primary health care networks. The district is the most natural administrative level promoted by the WHO for health delivery. Each district is small enough for the staff to understand the major problems and constraints of socio-economic and health development, yet large enough to develop the technical and managerial skills essential for planning and management (Tarim, 1991). In the Iranian health network, the executive units at district level are the health house, rural and urban health centres, rural health worker (*Behvarz*) training centre, district health centre, and district hospital. All of these function under the directorate of the District Health Network.

Health centres

The rural health centre *(Markaz e Behdaasht e Roostaaei)*, is a village-based facility that supervises the health affairs in its own and a number of other cealth couses in neighbouring villages. On average, each rural health centre covers the health needs of about 9000 people, and there are about 2000 functioning rural health centres in the country. Apart from a physician, the staff of a fully established rural health centre includes technicians for family health, disease control, environmental health, oral health, laboratory, nurse aid(s) and administrative personnel. All the staff function under the doctor's leadership. The rural health centres provide out-patient care and case finding among patients referred from health houses. They advise health houses on monitoring and follow-up. They supervise activities in the areas of family health, disease control, and environmental health. They offer oral health services, participate in health projects and support their assigned health houses in their needs. They also have certain mental health responsibilities that will be discussed later.

Health houses

The health house (*Khaneh e Behdasht*) is the grass root health facility in the rural areas. Each health house is capable of serving about 1500 people, though it is by no means an inflexible limit. There are about 15,000 such health houses in the country with about 28,000 *Behvarzes* working in them. Many Iranian villages have populations of less than 1500. Therefore, to ensure cost-effectiveness, each health house covers one or more satellite villages as well as its main village. The distance between the main village and each satellite village is defined as being no more than one hour's walk. Each health house has one (or more) male and one (or more) female health workers (*Behvarz*). Each Behvarz comes from the same village they will be stationed in later. The main function of a health house is to offer primary health care services to the community it serves. A well-established health house has some other tasks. These include annual health census, public education, a wide range of family health activities including immunisation, family planning, disease control, as well as some well-defined mental health tasks. The following is how one of the people who has devised the Iranian health system has summarised the important role of Health Houses: 'The Health House . . . effectively bridges a serious gap that persisted in Iran right up to the expansion of Primary Health Care (PHC) networks. Before this versatile health care facility was created, the provision of services to the most deprived rural communities on the scale and of the quality now attained, was neither feasible, nor conceivable.' (Shadpour, 1994) As in many other parts of the world, provision of health services to the urban areas has not been easy or straightforward. There are different and competing private, semi-private and governmental health providers in the city, so that bringing them together under one umbrella is impossible. Even in the government sponsored networks, urban areas lack a grass root facility like health houses. It is only recently that some innovative ideas are being developed to find a replacement for this community-based system. These include the use of different volunteer neighbourhood groups, among which the ones connected to 'Healthy City' projects are gaining importance. The official equivalent of the rural health centre in the cities is the Urban Health Centre (*Markaz e Behdaasht e Shahri*), which performs the same type of functions for a population of 12,000. There are about 2000 such centres in the country. All medical students spend a part of their training in different levels of primary health care (PHC) fields.

As a result of the implementation of the above health system in Iran, infant mortality rate has dropped from 145 per thousand live births in 1960 to 28 per thousand live births in 1997, and is steadily decreasing. Major infectious and nutritional diseases are controlled. The rate of vaccination for common childhood infections (designated by WHO as *Extended Programme of Immunisation (EPI) target diseases*) is above 95%. Overall life expectancy is 69 years, compared with 57 years in 1979, and total fertility rate is down from 6 in 1974 to 2.6 in 1996.

MENTAL HEALTH

General considerations

Mental health and care of psychiatric patients were, until the late 1970s, provided through traditional psychiatric hospitals. A few such facilities existed in different parts of the country and offered traditional, mainly in-patient services to those who could reach them. No concept of comprehensive mental health services existed and no facility could be found outside a few large cities and metropolitan areas. The first university psychiatric ward was opened in a general hospital belonging to Tehran university in the 1940s. In the early 1950s this ward was moved to Roozbeh Hospital and it became the first teaching psychiatric hospital in the country. The idea of community mental health was introduced for the first time in the mid 1970s. Then, the newly established Society for Rehabilitation of the Disabled started to designate catchment areas and develop outpatient treatment through community mental health centres. Simultaneously, new comprehensive mental health centres were built in different parts of the country, and the returning of treated patients to the community started. Many of these efforts continued after the revolution through the newly established Tehran Psychiatric Institute. This institute was the main technical adviser of the Ministry of Health when the implementation of the Iranian National Mental Health Programme started in the mid 1980s.

The country has about 600 psychiatrists. The distribution of these psychiatrists is still not ideal. Tehran and a number of other large cities get a disproportionate number of psychiatrists. This uneven distribution was worse in the past. However, in recent years, through a series of regulations and the introduction of certain incentives, more specialists including psychiatrists are being attracted to work in deprived areas of the country. Therefore, nowadays, psychiatrists practice in all the provinces and many districts. Psychiatry is being taught as an independent subject in all medical schools, and all the students have mandatory clinical psychiatric training. Policies regarding internship in psychiatry differ in different universities, but it is mandatory for one month only in some universities. Curricula of medical schools contain mental health and community psychiatry subjects, but there is resistance for more change. There are 10 psychiatric residency programmes in the country. Together, they have a total of more than 100 resident psychiatrists under training. One programme (in Shaheed Beheshti University of Medical Sciences) offers subspeciality training in child psychiatry. Certification is undertaken by a national board through an examination consisting of written, verbal and clinical aspects.

The utilisation of general (Bachelor of Science) psychologists in mental health services started before the revolution, during the time that psychiatric services were being reformed by the Society for the Rehabilitation of the Disabled. Postgraduate training in clinical psychology started in the early 1970s and first degrees (of Master of Science in Clinical Psychology) were awarded by Tehran university. After the revolution new programmes for both M.Sc. and Ph.D. started in Tehran Psychiatric Institute, and there are now four programmes awarding the degree of Master of Science in clinical psychology. An M.Sc degree for psychiatric nursing exists and mental health subjects are included in the curriculum of all nursing schools. The country has schools for occupational therapy and social work. Recently an M.Sc. degree for psychiatric occupational therapy has been introduced.

In the area of research, the first serious epidemiological studies were done by Bash and Bash (Liechti, 1987) during the 1950s. Other research activities were initiated by Davidian. (Davidian, Izadi, Nehapetian, & Motabar, 1971) During the 8 years' war with Iraq a number of studies were also undertaken on different aspects of war-related mental health problems and PTSD. During recent years a qualitatively new era in research has started, characterised by the institutionalisation of research in the work of an increasing number of post-graduate students. This is shown in a better quality of theses, and by improved supervision. However, research still has a long way to go and one major obstacle is a low degree of familiarity and emphasis on foreign language, and a low level of access to major global centres of research.

National mental health programme

The drafting of the national mental health programme of Iran took place in 1985, in collaboration with the WHO. The programme was then offered for approval, which it received in 1986. It was also the result of a joint effort, in which the Ministry of Health and three universities of Iran, Mash'had and Tehran were involved. The group was convened by the Tehran Psychiatric Institute.

The objectives of the programme are as follows:

1. To make basic mental health services available to all the people in the Islamic Republic of Iran in the near future. The emphasis would be on the most vulnerable and deprived groups in urban and rural areas who, so far, have not received any services, especially ones living in remote areas.
2. To produce a model of mental health services compatible with the social and cultural structure of Iranian society and encourage community participation in building mental health services.
3. To increase people's knowledge and skills of mental health in the service of improving general health. To encourage the people in the direction of wider use of mental health principles in order to promote health. To accelerate socio-economic development and improve the quality of life.
4. To plan appropriately for provision of necessary mental health care for all who have in one way or another suffered mentally during the current war.* (i.e. the refugees, the homeless, the disabled, the bereaved, and the mentally ill), and to plan for long-term services needed to face the consequences of this war in the future.

The main strategy of this national programme is Integration of mental health into the primary health care system, through a set of strategic actions in the areas of services, training and administration. Division of labour based on a clear understanding and definition of Levels is another principle of this programme.

At the level of health house (health post in the cities), the multipurpose health worker (*Behvarz* in the villages and volunteer in the cities) is given the following tasks:

1. Alertness to the presence of mental and psychological symptoms and complaints as health problems.

* At the time of drafting and approval of the National Programme of Mental Health, the Iran–Iraq war was fiercely being fought and war related issues had highest priority. In a revision of the national programme that is scheduled to take place in 1998–99, such emphasis could be placed on provision of care for victims of all stressful conditions and disasters.

2. Understanding and ability to diagnose four common conditions of minor mental illness, major mental illness, mental retardation and epilepsy.
3. Referral to the GP and receiving back referrals for follow-up.
4. Enough familiarity with psychiatric treatments (i.e. medications and their major side-effects), for the purpose of follow up.
5. Common understanding of stress-related conditions and simple stress reduction methods. Also having some knowledge regarding the effects of psychological factors on physical illnesses and vice versa particularly in vulnerable groups like adolescent, children, pregnant women, and the elderly.

At the level of health centre, the GP is in charge of the following tasks:

1. Receiving referrals from the health houses and/or volunteers.
2. Familiarity with major psychiatric conditions and their treatments with particular emphasis on common psychiatric illnesses. Initiation of drug and supportive treatment for psychosis, epilepsy, depression, and severe anxiety states, with required knowledge of the drugs and their effects and side-effects.
3. Referring those cases that need specialist's intervention to clinics and hospitals.
4. Supervision of the work of family health and disease control technicians.

A disease control technician of the health centre supervises the health workers (*Behvarz*) in case finding and referral. She or he also helps the GP regarding referrals and back referrals, and keeps the statistics.

The duties of the family health technician are:

1. Supervision of the health workers in establishing supportive relations with the families and the community.
2. Training of the *Behvarz* in areas of school mental health, problems of mothers and children and simple preventive measures.
3. Mental health education for the community and family alone with the Behvarz.

Supervision for the work of rural and urban health centres is provided by the psychiatrist or a specially trained GP who is connected to the district health centre. The programme envisages that each district general hospital would at least have five psychiatric beds. This aim has not been achieved in most hospitals.

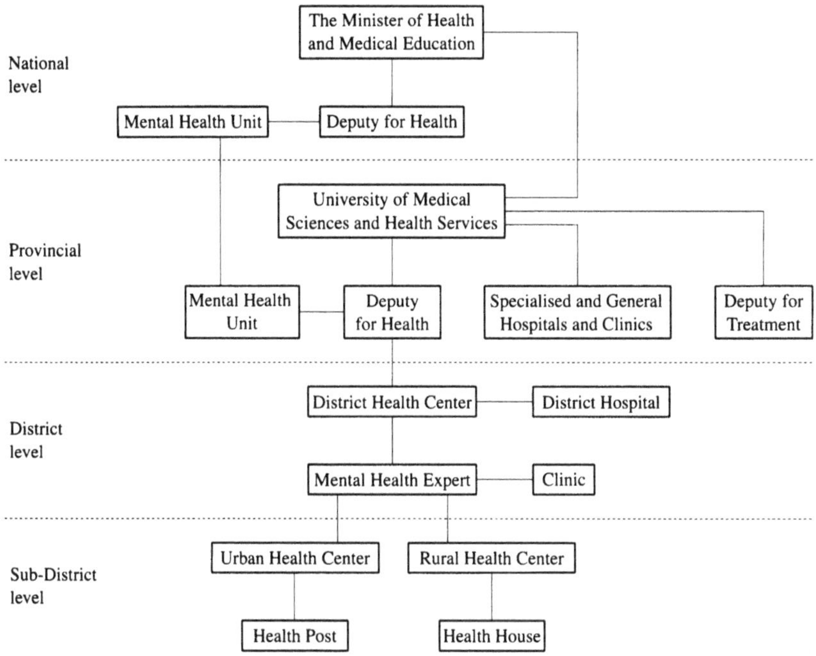

FIG. 11.2. The chart shows the organisational scheme for the implementation of the Iranian national mental health programme.

Higher level supervision is being provided at provincial level through universities of medical sciences and at national level through directorate general for disease control. Technical guidance for this directorate comes from the national Mental Health Advisory Committee.

The Integration of Mental Health into Primary Health Care System started as two pilot projects in districts of *Shahreza* and *Shahr i Kurd* in 1987 (Shahmohammadi, 1990). Since then it has been continuously going on and growing in all parts of the country; (Bolhari & Mohit, 1996; WHO, 1988, 1990) and during these years, additional features and innovations in areas like school and urban mental health have been added to it (WHO, 1993, 1995). At present the programme is active at least in one district in each of the country's 28 provinces. In a number of provinces such activities exist in all districts. Throughout the country, 2998 health houses and 914 rural health centres are active in this area. More than 6000 *Behvarzes* and 2000 GPs have been trained. (WHO, 1997) Although the integration in urban areas lags behind, it is hoped that with approaches like the one in Tehran and a similar one in Isfahan it would become possible to help it flourish.

The mental health activities in Iran have been visited and evaluated by different international experts. An official evaluation was done in 1995 by world level experts. The results of this evaluation clearly show the success of the programme in general. The evaluation also is mindful of the shortcomings and the problems the programme may face in the future. It has given a set of recommendations for future expansion. It cautions against burn-out syndrome of field personnel and questions related to sustainability (Sartorius, Wig, Murthy, Bertolotte, & Mohit, 1995).

The city of Tehran's mental health services

The city of Tehran uses the services of 300 psychiatrists, about 2600 psychiatric beds, 4 government psychiatric hospitals and 3 psychiatric wards in general hospitals. Two child psychiatry services exist that are connected to the universities. Five private psychiatric hospitals are also active in the city. The services for people with learning disability and the elderly are provided both through welfare organisations and the private sector. A number of private Tehran hospitals offer residency programmes of psychiatry, one centre offers a fellowship programme in child psychiatry.

The major psychiatric hospital is a classically huge institution (1700 beds) called Razi Psychiatric Centre. It is located in the southern suburbs of Tehran in a working class neighbourhood and is surrounded by two cement factories. It is being run by a welfare organisation. Its general condition is clean and reasonably well kept, the basic needs of patients are met well, medications and other treatment modalities are available—but the philosophy that governs it is institutionalisation. Up to now, all efforts to break it into smaller units scattered in different parts of the city have been unsuccessful. In the past this hospital was offering services to many parts of the country, but in recent years almost all the country's provinces have some psychiatric facility, and the reliance on this hospital for other parts of the country has decreased. It has some affiliation with different universities and some teaching and research activities are conducted there.

Other psychiatric hospitals and wards in general hospitals mainly belong to the universities of medical sciences. Among the university hospitals, mention should be made of Roozbeh Hospital which is the oldest teaching psychiatric hospital in Iran, and perhaps in the Middle East. The army, navy, air force, police and national bank have their own psychiatric services. There is a widespread network of school mental health activities that mainly focus on prevention and promotion. A special out-patient service exists for university students.

Services for drug abuse are all under government control. Addiction is regarded as a criminal act and addicts are admitted to facilities supervised by the police. Recently, the welfare organisation in collaboration with the Ministry of Health and Central Bureau to Combat Addiction, have started new programmes in this area. Preventive activities exist through schools, media and 'Healthy City Projects'.

THE WHO HEALTHY CITIES PROJECTS

Healthy Cities is the name of an environmental health initiative of the WHO. The projects with this name aim towards continuous promotion and improvement of different aspects of health in urban settings through conscious, direct, and volunteer involvement of the people and intersectoral collaboration at national and local levels. The concept was introduced in Iran in 1990. The initial project started in one of the most deprived areas of south Tehran in February 1992. As the first activity of this project, the needs and expectations perceived by the people were collected through group discussion with 160 people selected through a systematically randomised sample of all the family files existing in the area's Urban Health Centre. These persons were invited to attend a meeting for discussion of the needs of their neighbourhood. They were divided into 10 groups, and each group was given the task of identifying what they would expect the Healthy City Project to do for them. Their suggestions and expectations were then systematically classified. It was based on these suggestions that the following seven committees were formed to plan and implement the programmes: General health; Education; Urban services; Employment and income generation; Sport; Community participation; and Mental health.

The committees started to meet at least once a week to plan, and then to implement, a range of activities in their respective areas. The following are some highlights:

General health committee. Experts from the Ministry of Health and Medical Education plus a number of community representatives are members of this committee. The most successful programme of this committee is The Health Volunteers. These volunteers are mainly women who are known in the neighbourhood to be sociable, intelligent, and ready to assist other people. Their duties are very similar to the duties of *Behvarz* in rural areas, and include issues like vaccination, breast feeding, control of diarrhoea, family planning, and selected environmental health activities. It is through the same volunteers that a part of mental health services is also provided. Use of volunteers has been an innovative approach that could fill a great existing gap in provision of health to urban dwellers, the gap that was filled in the villages by *Behvarz*.

Education committee. The members of the education committee are experts from the Ministry of Education, teachers of different levels from the community, university students living in the community and a number of interested persons. One of their most successful programmes has been School Health Volunteer *(Behdaashtyaar e madreseh.)*. These volunteers' students are interested in health activities and are trained to function as health agents in the school and community. The activities of these students have been observed by a group of WHO consultants who evaluated mental health programmes in Iran in 1995. The following is quoted from them: The first thing that greeted us was the bright and clean school environment. Soon, we were met by well dressed, cheerful young girls. They were keen to share their activities. Initially they presented their work focusing on their different committees for health, school environment, nutrition, etc. On inquiry, they shared how their own attitudes and actions, along with that of their family members have changed due to the school health initiative. The aspect that remained with us, of the visit, was how well health-related matters were integrated into the educational life and the value of such an approach. The beneficiaries are the children and the citizens of the city.'

Urban services committee. Members include experts in urban development, city planning, architecture, environmental health, traffic management, green spaces, and a number of interested people from the neighborhood. They work in close collaboration with schools and other community resources. This committee needs serious coordination because at times it deals with opposing views and interests. This committee's activities include making the streets user-friendly for the disabled, and beautification of neighbourhoods and schools. Comprehensive planning for protection of green spaces and public parks and gardens by the community is among their other activities.

Committee for employment and income generation. Experts from welfare organisations, Ministries of Labour and Education and some members of the community are among the members of this committee. They have been active in finding the cases of unemployment, provision of training, and finding proper jobs for many of them.

Committee for sport activities. Members are from the National Organisation for Sport and interested community and neighbourhood volunteers. They have been able to build sporting facilities and organise regular matches among 18 football teams competing for the Healthy City Cup.

Committee for Mental Health. This is an innovative committee of the Healthy City Project in Tehran. The activities of this committee will be described in detail in this chapter.

Mental health component of Healthy Cities Project in Tehran

As has already been described, the national mental health programme of Iran was more successfully implemented in rural areas. One of the main reasons for the difference between the two areas was the lack of first level support in urban settings. Healthy City Project and Neighbourhood Health Volunteers provided an alternative.

The Tehran Mental Health in Healthy City initiative is based on the recognition of the following:

1. Vast needs.
2. Poor utilisation of available services.
3. Need for focused and involved participation of the community.
4. Relatively limited resources.
5. Existing potential of the people to act as agents for change, as shown in other activities coordinated by Healthy City project.
6. Strong feeling that new solutions are possible through community involvement.
7. Willingness of the authorities to participate and help.

The above issues were creatively addressed by active involvement of the people in the programmes. The general population became active partners rather than passive recipients. By making mental health a people's programme, not only do all mental health needs get attention, but also the programmes do not become highly dependent on institutions and scarce high level professionals. A community then gets an opportunity to plan for better utilisation of these professionals. There is also greater scope for prevention of mental illnesses and promotion of mental health.

Objectives. The main objective of the programme is to provide the necessary mental health services to urban, suburban and slum dwellers; by using the possibilities of Healthy City Projects including Neighbourhood Health Volunteers. Specific objectives are:

1. Promotion and increase in knowledge and attitude of urban and suburban dwellers regarding mental health.
2. Improving the attitude of people living in the cities and suburban areas towards psychiatric illnesses through continuous mental health education.
3. Case finding for neuro-psychiatric illnesses.
4. Proper and timely intervention in the areas of treatment, and follow-up for the cases found through the system.
5. Active delivery of mental health services in the areas covered by each project.

Administrative strategies.

1. Formation of a mental health committee composed of the chief, district health centre, a consultant psychiatrist functioning as the main scientific and administrative adviser, psychologist, the officer responsible for preventive medicine, a representative from a welfare organisation and representatives from the community based on their interest, willingness and possibilities to assist.
2. The establishment of health posts (*paaigaah e behdaashti*): Health posts in the cities would replace health houses in the villages. Such posts are being established in relation to urban health centres, mosques, professional societies and other volunteer organisations and each of them covers a population of approximately 10,000 people. The health posts are the centre of activity of the volunteers. Each volunteer provides a defined number of health services, some related to mental health, to a part of this population in 30–50 families.
3. Each health post is administered by one of the volunteers. She functions as the guide and coordinator for others and maintains the link between the volunteers and their responsible officer in the urban health centre.
4. The establishment of a referral system. Such a system would provide referral from the community (where family, teachers and health volunteers are), to the Urban Health Centre (where the GP is). It also makes provision for referral to and from the district mental health clinic and psychiatric centres (where specialist resources and services are).
5. Constant supervision of all levels.

Division of work. The duties of GPs, experts and technicians are the same as the ones described for the rural areas. The volunteer's duties also have many similarities to the *Behvarz*. However, they concentrate more on the living conditions of the chronic patients. They effectively become involved in decreasing institutionalisation by constant contact with the patients, families and the community.

Training and research. The following formal training activities are being done in connection with the programme:

1. Preparation of training manuals for volunteers and GPs.
2. Attracting GPs interest through holding on the job training courses mainly by using the training material based on ICD–10/PHC.
3. Training and orientation courses for different levels of urban health personnel particularly disease control and family health technicians. The aim of such training is to make them ready to supervise the volunteers, form files for the cases that are found, and prepare reliable statistics.
4. Continuing training of volunteers (strictly according to the prepared text), by the technicians and under supervision of a district mental health adviser.

The whole programme covers four Healthy City projects in and around Tehran. In each of these projects a municipal zone collaborates with one university of medical sciences for the implementation of the project. A total of 16 physicians, 21 mental health experts, 11 technicians and 182 volunteers is involved in this stage of the project. General practitioners go through a three day training given by the psychiatrist in charge of mental health in the concerned university. Another three day training course is designed for technicians. This course is conducted by mental health experts of the university. Finally a 20 session training course is designed for the volunteers and is given by the technicians.

The following studies are being done as the project progresses:

1. Attitude and knowledge test of the community. Two hundred tests and 200 control questionnaires will be filled in each of the four regions, making it a total of 1600 questionnaires.
2. Attitude and knowledge test of volunteers before training programme in test and control groups.
3. A prevalence study based on 800 case finding questionnaires. A total of 800 questionnaires will be filled. A 2-day training course is held for the technicians who fill the questionnaire.
4. The number of patients in in-patient facilities whose addresses are from these areas is determined. This number will be checked periodically to determine the impact of this programme.
5. The attitude and knowledge tests of the volunteers and the community will be repeated in one and two years.

Promotion of mental health and prevention of mental illness. The mental health related activities in Tehran are not only directed towards physical structures, case finding and mental illnesses. There are many community-based activities which are in one way or another effective in inducing a better atmosphere for people to live, and thus promote mental health.

The following mental health promotion and prevention activities have been undertaken:

1. Formation of health committees in the schools in the areas covered by the WHO Healthy City Project. These committees are specifically effective in promotion of healthy life styles and the prevention of phenomena like addiction.
2. Building of many smaller neighbourhood cultural centres in different parts of the city, particularly in deprived areas. These centres provide different groups of citizens access to many cultural and scientific activities, thus promoting good and positive mental health.
3. Introduction of vocational training for women, which has proved tremendously effective in giving women from deprived urban communities new opportunities with potentially positive effects on the prevention of depression.

DISCUSSION AND FUTURE CHALLENGES

National programme of mental health

The important feature of the mental health program in Iran is the realisation of integration of mental health into primary health care system on a national scale. The experience of Iran started as one of the pioneer experiments of its kind in the eastern Mediterranean region of the World Health Organisation. However, this programme was not by any means the first of its kind. Outside the region, India had started such a programme many years ago. Pakistan and Egypt also started the programme earlier than Iran. Why could it become a nationwide programme in Iran? In this connection, it is notable that the WHO published the landmark publication *Introduction of a Mental Health Component into Primary Health Care* years after most of these experiences, and it was undoubtedly influenced by them.

The main factor in favour of national level expansion of the Iranian programme has been the existence of a very well supported, culturally acceptable primary health care system. The fact that basic human resources *(Behvarzes)* of this system are chosen from the village people is a very important factor. Other reasons may be found in true political will behind the whole health network. Undoubtedly, the existence of a number of mental health professionals willing and ready to challenge the old system with the idea of integration of mental health into primary health care has also played a role. The support and understanding of a considerable part of the psychiatric community have also played an important role. The formal WHO evaluation has shown that the success of this programme in Iran is real. The same group have also cautioned about the need to safeguard the sustainability of this programme. Continuous supervision, training and research are needed to ensure the realisation of such an objective. In order to safeguard the continuation of such a success there is also a need to ensure that all levels get some kind of incentive and compensation for their interest and labour. Continued support from psychiatric and other professional communities is also necessary.

The present author also believes that the greatest future challenge of this programme is sustainability and facing the issue of burn-out syndrome. The experience of the past 10 years has shown that the weakest link in the chain of referrals is the health centre and where GPs work. In many countries, where in response to growing and unmet national needs a large number of GPs have been trained in a short span of time; difficulties of a different nature have arisen. In this connection, the main difficulties are in relation to the over-saturation of possibilities for working in large cities and reluctance of young physicians to work in small, rural areas. Many times, this unwillingness can be seen in form of decreased enthusiasm for work and indifference to new ideas and whatever they perceive an addition to their daily routine. Adding this to the fact that a GP working in a rural health centre usually has a busy practice, shows the necessity of paying serious attention to this issue. Although the same problem still does not apply to the *behvarzes*, one should always be alerted to the possibility of such a problem, and think ahead for finding solutions in the form of incentives, continuous training, and regular one-to-one supervision.

Healthy City and Volunteers Project

This is quite a new approach and it is still too early to speak about its success or failure. Need for reform of psychiatric services in greater Tehran has been felt in the last 25 years and some steps have been taken in this direction. Undoubtedly, there is still strong resistance that needs to be overcome. The success of integration of mental health into the primary health care network was a very important factor in bringing about positive attitudinal changes in decision makers, community and professionals. Mental health started to be seen as a real and applicable part of health, and innovative approaches started to be appreciated and accepted. This programme is not going to replace psychiatric services in Tehran, but, if successful, can function as a model for change. It uses a truly community-based approach, and can become a basis for a multisectoral model. Through such a model, mental health services in general, and the care of chronic mental patients in particular, can be provided. The Healthy City projects provide the organisational framework for integration of many health-related activities into the complex fabric of urban life. In such a set-up, care of patients becomes an integral part of a community work that has other programmes and horizons. Therefore, a gradual change of attitudes towards mental illness and patients for the better will ensue.

The constraints such a programme may face and challenges for the future come from different sources.:

1. As the programme is multisectoral, one area of concern is coordination between the sectors involved. The formation of committees with representation from different sectors is an important positive step to avoid conflicts of concerns and interest. So far as mental health is concerned, such a multisectoral committee should include representatives from the concerned health authority, nearest mental health unit or hospital, users or their representatives, schools, nearby cultural and sport centres, and sometimes police and the judiciary.
2. Difficulties may also arise from burn-out syndrome among the volunteers. This constitutes a problem for all areas of volunteer work. Refresher courses and different types of supervision, encouragement and moral and material incentives are necessary.
3. One challenge is objectively to demonstrate that the programme has an actual impact. Therefore, the programme needs a solid basis for constant evaluation and built-in research on different areas like impact on the pattern of hospitalisation and discharge, or pathways patients choose for getting help. Only through such an on-going evaluation would it become possible to recommend more widespread application of such an approach.
4. Finally, it is a reality that during the last few years, vast activities have been undertaken by the Ministry of Health and Medical Education at national level and Tehran municipality in the city. These activities have changed the major health indicators of the country as well as the face of the city that is now one of the cleanest in the Middle East. The country now has a comprehensive health network in which many programmes including mental health are integrated. The city has been enriched with many new gardens, cultural centres, museums, libraries and the like. To a certain extent, a whole new atmosphere of modernity and progress has prevailed. Such conditions also induce progress in many new areas, including better mental health and improved, decentralised services for the patients. This is a hope

shared by many and undoubtedly its full realisation would need constant work and vigilance.

ACKNOWLEDGEMENTS

The author is grateful to many people and particularly the community and Healthy City staff in south Tehran who were his main teachers. He also wishes to express deepest thanks to the following for their kind advice, support and useful information provided to him by them: Dr Ismail Akbari, I. R. Iran's Deputy Minister of Health and Medical Education at the time this persentation was being prepared; Mr Abbas Bagheri, Mental Health Unit, Ministry of Health and Medical Education; Dr Jaafar Bolhari, Director, Tehran Psychiatric Institute; Eng. Farajullahi, Director, Healthy City Project, South Tehran; Dr Javid Hashmi, World Health Organisation Representative in I.R. Iran; Eng. Honarbakhsh, Ms. Arbab'ha, Mr Omid Mohit, and their associates in Noghreh public relations company in Tehran for the great film they made to accompany this paper to London; Eng. Kumars Khoshchashm, Regional Adviser, Healthy City, Eastern Mediterranean Regional Office, World Health Organisation; Dr Fereydoun Mehrabi, Chairman, Department of Psychiatry, Iran University of Medical Sciences, Tehran Psychiatric Institute; Dr M.H. Niknam, Director General, international relations, Ministry of Health and Medical Education; Eng. Salmanmanesh, Senior adviser, Healthy City, Tehran; Dr Davood Shahmohammadi, Tehran Psychiatric Institute; Dr Ali Zojaji, Dieector, Mental Health, Ministry of Health and Medical Education.

REFERENCES

Bash, K.W. & Bash-Liechti, D. (1987). *Developing Psychiatry*, Berlin: Springer-Verlag.

Bolhari, D.J. & Mohit, A. (1996). *Integration of mental health into primary health care system in Hashtgerd (a suburb of Tehran). Final report of a research project.* Iran University of Medical Sciences (Tehran Psychiatric Institute). [Farsi (Persian)].

Davidian, H., Izadi, S., Nehapetian, V., & Motabar, M. (1971). A preliminary study of prevalence of psychiatric disorders in the Caspian sea area (Roodsar district) of Iran. *Behdaasht e Iran*, *3*, 145–156. [Farsi (Persian)].

Sartorius, N., Wig, N.N., Murthy, S.R., Bertolotte, J., & Mohit, A. (1995). *Independent Evaluation of Iranian Mental Health Program.* Alexandria: WHO Eastern Mediterranean Regional Office.

Shadpour, K. (1994). *Primary health care system in Iran.* Iran's Ministry of Health and Medical Education and UNICEF.

Shahmohammadi, D. (1990). *Comprehensive report of the pilot project of Integration of Mental Health into Primary Health Care System in* Shahr i Kurd *district of* Chahar Mahal va Bakhtiary *province.* Ministry of Health and Medical Education Tehran. [Farsi (Persian)].

Tarim, E. (1991). *Towards a Healthy District.* Geneva: World Health Organisation.

World Health Organisation (1988). *Report of the 'The Intercountry Meeting on Progress achieved in Mental Health Programs'*, Isfahan, I.R. Iran. WHO-EM/MENT/115–E. Alexandria: WHO Regional Office for the Eastern Mediterranean.
World Health Organisation (1990). *Report of 'The Second Intercountry Meeting on Progress achieved in National Mental Health Programs*, Nicosia, Cyprus, WHO-EM/MENT/116–E. Alexandria: WHO Regional Office for the Eastern Mediterranean.
World Health Organisation (1993). *Report of 'The Intercountry Consultation on School Mental Health'*. Islamabad, Pakistan, November 1993. WHO-EM/MNH/138–E/L. Alexandria: WHO Regional Office for the Eastern Mediterranean.
World Health Organisation (1995). *Report of 'Intercountry Meeting on The Evaluation of The Progress of National Mental Health Programs in The Eastern Mediterranean Region'*. Casablanca, Morocco, WHO-EM/MNH/142–E/L. Alexandria: WHO Regional office for the Eastern Mediterranean.
World Health Organisation (1997). *Draft report of Intercountry Meeting on Needs Assessment in Mental Health*. Tehran, I.R. Iran, September 7–11. Alexandria: WHO Regional Office for the Eastern Medioterranean.

CHAPTER TWELVE

Community-based mental health care in Verona, Italy

Michele Tansella, Francesco Amaddeo, Lorenzo Burti, Nicola Garzotto, and Mirella Ruggeri
Università di Verona, Italy

THE CITY OF VERONA, ITALY

Aim of chapter

The aim of this chapter is to describe the mental health care system of the City of Verona, Italy. The principles on which our system is organised will be briefly illustrated and some epidemiologically-based data, collected over the last 18 years using the South-Verona Psychiatric Case Register (PCR), will be presented. Finally the results of some evaluative studies conducted so far in our area will be summarised.

Verona and Italy

Italy is a country with a population of 56.8 million (67% classified as urban). The most densely populated parts of the country are in the north and there is a north–south split. Italy is rich in important library and art collections. Its economy is the fifth largest in the world and is based on industry in the north and agriculture in the south, with substantial regional differences. Services account for more than half the gross national product.

In 1978 a National Health Service (NHS) providing free health care replaced the existing national insurance system. Life expectancy is 81 years and 74 years for females and males respectively (1995 data). Other information is reported in Table 12.1.

TABLE 12.1
Sociodemographic Characteristics of the City of Verona and of Italy

	City of Verona	*Italy*
Population*	255,824	56,778,031
Area (km^2)*	199.1	301,302
Mean population density*	1285.0	188.0
Age (per 100 total population)*		
under 15 years	12.1	15.8
15–64 years	70.1	68.8
65 years and over	17.8	15.4
Youth dependency ratio (1)*	17.2	23.1
Age dependency ratio (2)*	25.5	22.4
Dependency ratio (3)*	42.7	45.4
People living alone (per 100 total population)*	9.2	7.0
People without permanent address (per 100)**	0.2	N.K.
Birth rate (per 1K)***	8.0	9.2
Mortality rate (per 1K)***	10.4	9.6
Infant mortality rate (per 1K live births/yr)***	4.9	6.6
Mean No. of rooms/resident*	1.8	1.8
Households without bathroom (per 100 households)*	3.6	3.1
Employed population, by economic sector (per 100 all employed)*		
Agriculture	2.0	7.6
Industry	29.1	35.6
Services	68.9	56.7
Employed population, by sex*		
Males	70.9	63.7
Females	41.7	34.0
All	56.0	48.7
Unemployed population, by sex*		
Males	4.8	11.8
Females	4.8	9.7
All	4.8	10.7

(*) Based on the latest national Census, 1991 (ISTAT, 1994; 1995).
(**) Based on an estimate made by the *Comune di Verona* (*Comune di Verona*, 1996).
(***) Data referring to the City of Verona are taken from the *Annuario Statistico*, 1995 (*Comune di Verona*, 1996); those referring to Italy from the Italian Statistical Abstract, 1994 (ISTAT, 1996).
(1) Children under 15 years supported by each 100 population of the age group 15–65 years.
(2) Elderly over 65 years supported by each 100 population of the age group 15–65 years.
(3) Dependent persons (children under 15 years and elderly over 65 years) supported by each 100 population of the age group 15–65 years.

Verona. It is pleasant to live in Verona, a beautiful city with many noteworthy architectural landmarks. The town is a human size, and the people are friendly and open-minded, as well as strongly attached to local traditions. It can be seen from Table 12.1 that Verona, as compared with the whole country, has a lower birth rate and youth dependency ratio, a lower infant mortality rate, and a lower percentage of unemployed population, both for males and females. The employed population, for both sexes, is higher and more people are employed in services and less in the agriculture and in the industry sectors. Verona is predominantly middle class, with services and industry comprising 92.3% of the economic sector. It is a wealthy, university city, which has an airport and is an important rail and marketing centre. It manufactures textiles, machinery, paper, chemicals, processed food, and shoes.

HISTORY OF MENTAL HEALTH SERVICES IN ITALY AND IN VERONA

The 1978 reform that radically changed mental health care

The new mental health Act, law 180, passed in May 1978 by the Italian Parliament, replaced the existing law, which dated back to 1904. The new law was part of the legislation that introduced the National Health Service (NHS). The main provisions of the Italian psychiatric reform, which evolved from innovative services that took place in several cities between 1961 and 1978, under the influence of Professor Franco Basaglia, were the following:

1. It called for a gradual dismantling of all large mental hospitals by blocking new admissions to these institutions after 1978 and all admissions after 1982. Abrupt deinstitutionalisation of chronic in-patients has not occurred and state and private hospitals today continue to care for a consistently decreasing number of these hospital chronic patients. Complete closure of all mental hospitals is expected in Italy during 1998.
2. As a rule, treatment would be made available to mental patients in their own environment and community services would provide the full range of psychiatric interventions for specified geographical areas.
3. Hospitalisation, both voluntary and compulsory, would take place only in small units of no more than 15 beds, located in general hospitals and being part of the community-based services.
4. Procedures for involuntary commitment were carefully detailed to safeguard patients' civil rights.

The Italian model of deinstitutionalisation: closing the front door of mental hospitals while implementing 'alternative' instead of 'additional' community-based services

A key point for reaching the goal of reducing and closing mental hospital beds is the type of organisation of the new community-based services (Thornicroft & Tansella, in press). They can be either additional (also called complementary), or alternative to the mental hospital. These are actually two different ways of organising community-services. The former model allows back-up by the mental hospital, which survives as a place where the most difficult and refractory cases can still be admitted and stay for a long period of time; the latter explicitly calls for the closure of mental hospitals and for the replacement of the care they provide with that offered by decentralised, residential facilities as well as by other programmes, run by the community-based mental health service for all patients, including the most severely ill and most difficult to treat (Tansella & Zimmermann Tansella, 1988). Italy chose to divert patients to alternative community services thus reducing, and then eventually stopping admissions to mental hospital altogether. Thus the mental hospital population would slowly decline as long-term residents were discharged or died.

Mental health care in Verona before and after the 1978 reform

Before 1978 mental health care in Verona was centred on the mental hospital. A new state mental hospital of 760 beds, the last constructed in Italy, was completed in 1968 on the outskirts of Verona, 15 km from the city centre. This hospital, run in a traditional way, had very few links with the community either in terms of structures or staff.

In 1970 an Academic Department of Psychiatry was opened, as part of a new school of medicine. Until 1978 the role of this department, as of any other university psychiatric department in the country, was mainly that of conducting research and providing training to medical and post-graduate students as well as psychiatric care to patients selected according to ill-defined criteria and psychiatric psychological consultations for other departments of the 1200 bed academic general hospital. It was not dealing with patients compulsorily admitted (who had to be admitted to the mental hospital), or with long-term chronic patients, or with rehabilitation, day care or home visits.

As the department developed, the principles and the practice of community care became the main topic of interest for most members of the staff. New research projects on social and epidemiological aspects of mental illness started (Tansella & Williams, 1989), so after the approval of the new law in 1978 the Department of Psychiatry of the University of Verona was the first academic department in Italy that accepted the proposal of the regional authorities to provide a comprehensive Community-based Mental Health Service (CMHS) for the entire adult population of a geographically-defined area, called South-Verona, with a population of 74,500. It is a predominantly urban area, with a population density of 1795/km^2 in the urban sector. Three other CMHSs, run by NHS staff, were set up for the remainder of the Province of Verona. Within the University Department of Psychiatry a psychiatric case register (PCR) was set up and the South-Verona CMHS was linked with a research unit for conducting evaluative research projects (Tansella, 1991). In 1987 the department was designated by the World Health Organization as a WHO Collaborating Centre for Research and Training in Mental Health and Service Evaluation.

THE SOUTH-VERONA COMMUNITY-BASED MENTAL HEALTH SERVICE (CMHS)

General organisation

The South-Verona Community-based Mental Health Service (CMHS) was designed as a unitary service, in which great emphasis is given to communication between all staff members and to integration between the various clinical activities.

All staff members are divided into three multidisciplinary teams, each serving a subsector of the South-Verona catchment area. A fourth smaller team provides a consultation and liaison service to the other departments of the academic general hospital.

The three main teams are organised according to a 'single staff module': with the exception of nurses, all staff work both inside and outside hospital and remain responsible for the same patients across different components of the service and through the different phases of treatment. There are hospital nurses (who cover the three round-the-clock shifts in the general hospital ward), hostel nurses, mental health centre nurses and community nurses (who cover two shifts, from 8 a.m. to 8 p.m., and are on call, two at a time, during the weekends and over night). Among nurses, only the community nurses are assigned to one of the three teams.

This module was designed to ensure continuity of care, both longitudinal continuity (through the different phases of treatment) and cross-sectional continuity (through the different components of the service). Within each team each patient is assigned to one particular member of the staff (case manager). Case managers may be doctors, psychologists or senior nurses.

Patients seen only at the out-patient department, by a psychiatrist or a psychologist, do not have a case manager (Tansella, 1991).

Principles of intervention

It is widely accepted that institutionalisation, especially if repeated or prolonged, facilitates and sometimes creates chronicity. One of the main aims of the new service was therefore to prevent or reduce hospitalisation, giving high priority to crisis intervention and long-term community-based care.

The style of intervention is psychosocial: the service aims to provide prompt, adequate and coherent answers to patients' needs, psychological and social as well as practical, while trying to decrease and control symptoms. Special emphasis is given to integrating different interventions, such as medication, family support, and social work. Case management, patient advocacy, and welfare provision are key aspects of these interventions.

Special attention is paid to the most disabled and difficult to manage, as well as to chronic patients: apart from the case manager, two or three other staff members are assigned to each patient, so that one is available at any given time, in spite of turnover, shifts and leave. These patients are regularly assessed and treatment plans are revised accordingly.

The evaluation of users' needs is routine in South-Verona, and the commitment to meeting them well established. Over the years, the service has acquired considerable resources and services to meet such needs. New types of worker have entered the scene: the *educatore professionale* (counsellor), the *operatore di assistenza* (support care provider), the *assistente domiciliare* (housekeeper). The emerging keystone of designing effective and efficient clinical work is matching existing programmes and individual needs, i.e. tailoring individual treatment plans by using all the resources already available.

Residential care in the community for long-term patients

Since the front door of the mental hospital was partially closed from 1978 and completely closed from 1982 an important aspect of our community-based service has been the provision of residential care for long-term patients. Two residential facilities are available in South-Verona, as part of the CMHS. One is a 24-hour-staffed supervised hostel, opened in 1990, with seven places for users in need of continuous supervision. It consists of two apartments in a block: a large one for the hostel proper, and a small adjoining one, used as a base by the staff. The other, a group home, also located in a normal block, provides 6–hour staff supervision on working days, and offers four places.

Each facility is coordinated by an *educatore* (counsellor), assisted by two *operatori di assistenza* (support care provider) per shift. Community nurses visit daily to administer medication and are on call overnight and on weekends for medical and psychiatric emergencies. The psychiatrist in charge of the mental health centre ensures medical supervision. Goals of the programme in both facilities are to provide accommodation, care, supervision, and rehabilitation in daily living and social skills to the residents.

Residents graduating from the supervised hostel may move to the group home, while those of the group home may move on to independent living. Alternatively, in order to prevent dislocation, a plan is under discussion of gradually withdrawing staff supervision and assigning the flat of the group home to the residents themselves, who will eventually assume full responsibility for it. Instead of displacing residents, the service will move out to start another group home elsewhere. Both facilities are funded by the ULSS (the local health authority) and residents are not required to contribute in any way, except for recreational activities and vacations. The ULSS also funds individual apartments assigned to long-term patients.

While all existing places are usually occupied and the need for more is voiced from time to time, the service aims to use this kind of facility sparingly (12 places in total, corresponding to a rate of about 16 per 100,000 at risk), and in preference to promote the preservation of independent living arrangements through community care and rehabilitation.

Communication within the CMHS and links with other health and social services

To ensure good communication and coordination between all staff members, a series of meetings take place: each day starts with a half-hour general meeting at the mental health centre. The doctor who has been on call for the previous day briefly reports on patients seen at the casualty department, and gives relevant information on all other patients who were referred to the service. The head nurses of the psychiatric ward in the hospital and of the mental health centre, one representative member of the staff from the hostel, and eventually other attendees briefly report on information that they believe should be known by all other staff members. After the general meeting each multidisciplinary team meets to organise clinical activities for the day, to be carried out in the various facilities of the service, including the hospital ward as well as community services. There are also weekly meetings on the hospital ward, at the mental health centre, at the hostel and meetings to discuss special cases.

The South-Verona CMHS is well integrated between ward and community, and allows patients easy access to most of its components and easy transfer from one component to another, according to needs. A drop-in approach is encouraged at the mental health centre and patients can seek care from specialist services directly, without previously attending GPs. However most patients are referred by GPs and referred back to them by the CMHS, when it is felt that less stigmatising care can be provided in primary care. There are good relations between primary and secondary care and meetings are held at regular intervals with GPs most interested to discuss how to improve the interface between primary care and mental health services. Our CMHS does not include services to schools, and liaison with police is only occasional.

Components of the CMHS

The community mental health centre is the linchpin of the CMHS. It is located in an old two-storey house with a garden, not far away from the academic general hospital, is open on weekdays from 8 a.m. to 8 p.m. and on Saturday from 8 a.m. to 5 p. m. Therapeutic programmes include crisis intervention, day care for acute and chronic patients and social skills groups. The centre also serves as an informal meeting place for users, and it is conceived as a flexible tool whose organisation can be modified from time to time to meet the user's changing needs.

The psychiatric ward is an open ward of 16 beds located in the academic general hospital which has about 1000 beds. It is a traditional hospital ward, similar to all other medical wards in the hospital and its door is locked when there are patients who have been compulsorily admitted.

The out-patient department provides psychiatric consultations and individual and family therapy. Offices are located in the general hospital and in the mental health centre.

The consultation liaison service for other medical and surgical departments maintains psychiatric integration with other hospital-based medical activities and ensures continuing contact with our patients when hospitalised for medical reasons.

There is a psychiatric emergency room service at the general hospital, open 24 hours a day, 7 days a week. It is run by a psychiatrist from our team, who is on call. To ensure therapeutic continuity, the doctor is usually assisted during working hours by the treatment team members who are (or will be) in charge of the patient requiring the urgent intervention. There is also an emergency night and weekend service, run by two psychiatric nurses from our team, who are on call and may provide care in our flats and in our hostel, as well as at our patients' homes, coordinated by the psychiatrist on call.

Home visits can be made to provide crisis intervention in response to emergency calls, but for chronic patients these are usually planned in advance and offer regular, long-term support and care to patients and their families with the goal of minimising relapses and hospital admissions. Home visits are highly regarded by the service and are well accepted by patients and families.

One group home and two apartments, offering different levels of supervision, and one hostel (with 7 beds, supervised 24 hours a day by support workers and counsellors and occasionally visited by nurses), are also available, as described above.

Staff

The South-Verona CMHS's permanent staff include 11 psychiatrists, 5 psychologists, 2 social workers, 3 health visitors, 13 community nurses, 14 ward nurses, and 2 counsellors. There are also a number of psychiatrists and psychologists in training, as well as *operatori di assistenza* (support workers) on contract. However, psychiatrists and psychologists, as well as other staff members, are involved not only in care of the patients, but also in research and teaching (for both undergraduate and post-graduate students and Ph.D. students).

In order to make comparisons with other services the average number of sessions (of approximately 4 hours) per week dedicated to clinical work has been estimated and corrected to that for a standard population of 100,000 adults (see Table 12.2).

Distinctive features of the mental health service in South-Verona

In conclusion, the main features of the South-Verona mental health service that could be considered distinctive to the service are as follows:

1. It is not experimental; we were set up as a result of legal changes based on a national Act. We have been running our services for 19 years.
2. It was designed and is still functioning as an alternative to the old hospital-based system of care, rather than being complementary to it. The front door of the mental hospital has been closed to new admissions since May 1978 and to all admission since January 1982.
3. The clinical model developed in South-Verona is systemic and is a single-staff module: all staff apart from nurses work both inside and outside hospital and remain responsible for the care of the same

TABLE 12.2
South-Verona Community Mental Health Service (CMHS) and Institute of Psychiatry of Verona: Number of Staff and Sessions (4 hours) of Staff Time per Week Dedicated to Clinical Work

	Number of Staff	*Sessions/week (Average)*	*Rate/100K adult pop.*
Professors of psychiatry	6	16	24.4
Psychiatrists	5	36	54.9
Trainee psychiatrists	20	120	183.1
Total	31	172	262.5
Professors of medical psychology	1	3	4.6
Psychologists	4	26	39.7
Trainee psychologists	4	24	36.6
Total	9	53	80.9
Social workers	2	16	24.4
Health visitors	3	12	18.3
Community nurses	13	117	178.6
Ward nurses	14	126	192.4
Operatori di assistenza (Hostel support care providers)	10	90	137.4
Educatori professionali (Hostel counsellors)	2	18	27.5

patients across different components of the service and through the different phases of care.

4. The South-Verona CMHS is well integrated, and allows easy and informal access to patients. It is a public service run by the National Health Service. Payment is not required, except for a fee for outpatient visits (this applies only to wealthy patients and for those who are not considered long-term).
5. Every effort is made to meet user's needs with individual care plans.
6. The evaluative research has included, since 1994, parallel evaluations of needs costs and outcome, as a way of monitoring and evaluating change.

OTHER PSYCHIATRIC SERVICES AVAILABLE TO SOUTH-VERONA RESIDENTS

Other psychiatric services within the larger province of Verona are available to South-Verona residents, as well as to residents of several other catchment areas. These include two private psychiatric hospitals (220 total beds), where patients from a larger area in north-east Italy can be admitted at the expense of the National Health Service, the state mental hospital of Verona (with 160 beds for old long-stay patients from the whole Province of Verona, admitted before 1982; on December 1995, 11 patients were from South-Verona and this is a very stable, low need group, who has any contact with our community-based service) and a private semi-residential facility for the rehabilitation of patients with learning disabilities, run by a charitable organisation. The mental hospital will be closed in April 1998 and the patients will be transferred to 24-hour staffed residential facilities. Verona is also served by a number of psychiatrists and psychologists in private practice (who are mainly involved in the treatment of minor psychiatric disorders), by a Centre for Substance Abuse (which has a larger catchment area) and by an out-patient psychiatric service for children and adolescents.

USER'S ORGANISATION

A self-help group was initiated in 1990 by a psychiatrist in training from the South-Verona Psychiatric Service and a few young mental health users. The group steadily grew to the present number of about 400 people in contact. In 1995 the group formed an association, *I Cavalieri di San Giacomo. San Giacomo* was the name of the old mental hospital in Verona.

The goals of the group are those typical of self-help organisations: participation is totally voluntary, the approach is non medical and involves reciprocal support, self-determination, counselling, education and advocacy. However, while other self-help groups have developed services completely outside the mental health system, this organisation operates within the system and in close collaboration with it. Three more goals are highly valued by the organisation and actively pursued through various activities: finding work and supporting those with jobs, housing, and education. Activities are many and various and take place every day of the week, especially in the evening and over weekends, when statutory services and other day care services are generally closed. During 1996 about 250 members have actually participated in one or more of the activities described above.

The self-help organisation has proven effective in both reducing personal and social discomfort and related stress, thus probably preventing the occurrence of some psychiatric episodes. By providing an alternative to professional care through reciprocal support, it has probably reduced the risk of institutionalisation. It has been far more effective than official bodies in helping users to find and maintain a job.

FROM SERVICE MONITORING TO SERVICE EVALUATION

The South-Verona psychiatric case register (PCR)

The South-Verona psychiatric case register (PCR) started on 31 December 1978 with a prevalence count and has been operating ever since. A detailed description of the case register has been reported elsewhere.

Clinical, administrative, and research uses of the PCR

The South-Verona PCR is used for clinical, administrative, and research purposes.

The clinical uses include:

1. The provision to the clinical teams of lists of severely mentally ill patients who have been in contact and are to be reassessed at regular intervals to ensure better continuity of care and improved practices. Working definitions of severely mentally ill can be reached pragmatically and are suggested to the register staff by the clinicians. For this purpose a combination of several variables, such as diagnosis, number of hospital admissions, number of episodes of illness, total number of contacts over a given period, occupational status, multiple agency use, and so on can be used.
2. The provision to the clinicians, on request, of a complete description of admissions and contacts of individual patients over a specified period of time.

Administrative uses of the register include:

1. The provision of prevalence figures, incidence rates, number of patients seen, and number of visits made over different periods of time.
2. The monitoring of the effects of changes in resources, organisation and needs, over time, and the use of the register as a basis for calculating direct costs of groups of patients (Amaddeo, Beecham, Bonizzato, Fenyo, Tansella, & Knapp, 1998).

Research uses are described below.

Longitudinal description of patterns of care, in-patient care before and after the reform, long-stay and long-term patients. Longitudinal monitor-

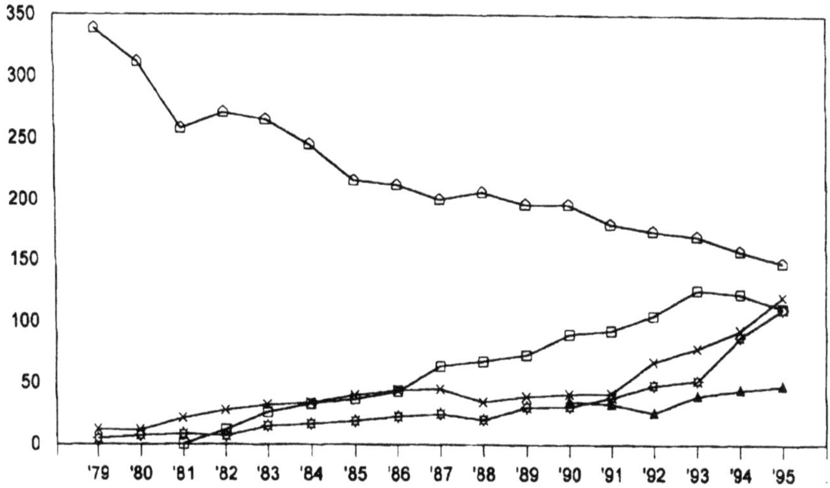

FIG. 12.1. Patterns of care (ratios per 1,000 adult South-Verona residents). ⊖ No. of days in hospital (acute and long-term); ∗ No. of home visits and other community contacts; ⊕ No. of days at days hospital and attendances at day centre; ⊟ No. of out-patient visits; ▲ No. of days in hostels.

ing of service utilisation in South-Verona showed that, from 1979 to 1995, hospital care (acute and long-term, provided by both public and private institutions) consistently decreased whereas out-patient care, home visits and other community contacts, number of days and attendance at day hospital and centres and number of days in the hostel run by the South-Verona CMHS steadily increased (see Fig. 12.1).

The decrease in the use of beds was mainly due to the decrease of long-stay patients in the state mental hospital and happened while psychiatric beds for short and medium-term stay were available (220 beds in private hospitals, where patients can be admitted at the expense of the National Health Service). Comparison of in-patient admissions before and after the 1978 psychiatric reform showed that in 1995 (17 years after the reform), as compared with 1977 (one year before), there was a 24% decrease of inpatient admissions, with a 94% decrease of compulsory admissions (which never exceed 22 admissions per 100,000 adult population) and a complete halt of admissions to state mental hospitals (Table 12.3). As a consequence the mean number of occupied beds per day consistently decreased over time and in 1995 was 62% lower than in 1977. This decrease is entirely due to the reduced number of patients remaining in the state mental hospital.

In 1995 the total number of beds occupied in both public and private

Table 12.3

In-Patient Admissions before (1977) and after the Psychiatric Reform (Ratios per 100,000 Adult South-Verona Residents)

	1977	*'79*	*'81*	*'83*	*'85*	*'87*	*'89*	*'91*	*'93*	*'95*	*Difference '95* vs. *'77*
Compulsory	55	8	10	18	8	22	22	11	11	3	−94%
To state mental hospitals (voluntary)	194	86	8	0	0	0	0	0	0	0	−100%
To other facilities:											
Public care	172	304	188	391	302	336	273	263	313	273	+59%
Private care	67	72	70	97	80	64	78	48	85	95	+43%
Total	488	469	277	507	390	422	373	321	509	371	−24%

Table 12.4

Mean Occupied Beds/Day before (1977) and after the Psychiatric Reform (Ratios per 100,000 Adult South-Verona Residents)

	1977	*'79*	*'81*	*'83*	*'85*	*'87*	*'89*	*'91*	*'93*	*'95*	*Difference '95* vs. *'77*
In state mental hospitals	86	69	50	40	32	29	29	25	19	17	−80%
In other public hospitals	9	16	12	17	17	16	15	16	15	16	+78%
In private hospitals	9	7	8	11	7	7	9	7	11	7	−22%
Total	104	93	71	68	57	52	53	48	46	40	−62%

hospitals was 40 per 100,000 adult South-Verona residents. If we exclude the state mental hospital the rate is 23 per 100,000 at risk and this latter figure has been constant for some years (Table 12.4).

We used the PCR to monitor chronic use of services over the years. Since, as a consequence of the Italian reform, admissions to mental hospitals have been halted and these are the main hospitals where patients admitted can become long-stay, we studied chronic use of services calculating rates of two groups of chronic patients: long-stay and long-term (who were not long-stay). Long-stay are defined as 'those who stay in one or more hospitals continuously for one year or more'. We defined as long-term 'those not-long-stay patients who were continuously in contact, for one year or more, with some psychiatric service (including psychiatric hospitals and wards), not necessarily the same service or only one service, with a period between two contacts never longer than 90 days'. Contacts here include a day in a psychiatric ward or in a day hospital or centre and all contacts with out-patient and domiciliary services.

Since 1979 the numbers of long-stay patients have been consistently decreasing, whereas the numbers of long-term patients steadily increased up to 1994, and for the first time showed a decrease in 1995 (Fig. 12.2). If we plot on a graph, every three years, new long-term patients, i.e. 'those who were not long-term (or in continuous care for one year or more) on triennial census days, but were long-term on subsequent annual census days' we can see that the first five cohorts showed a consistent

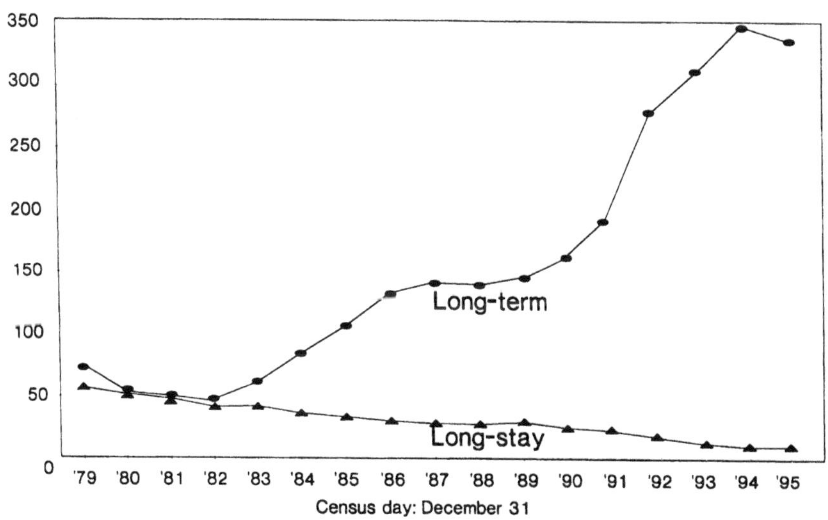

FIG. 12.2. Total long-stay and long-term patients (ratios per 100,000 adult South-Verona residents).

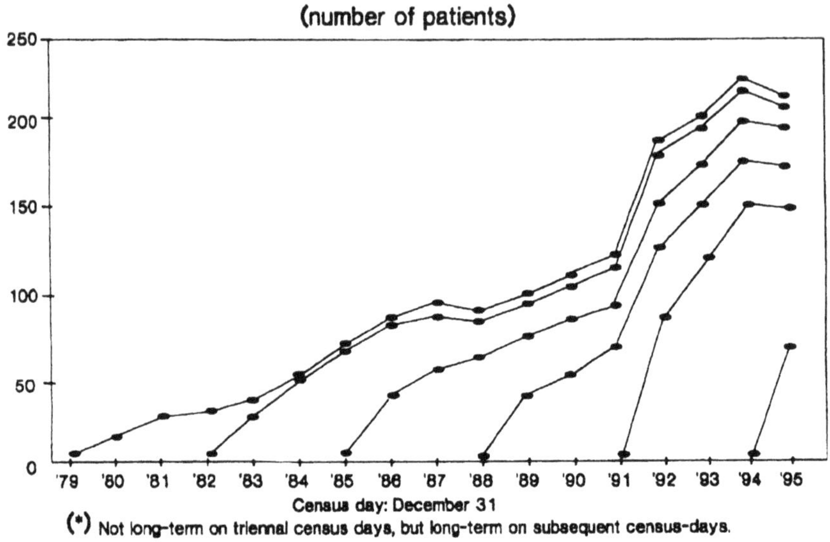

FIG. 12.3. Build-up in numbers of new long-term patients (not long-term on triennal census days, but long-term on subsequent census days).

accumulation of patients up to 1994 and that the sixth cohort, i.e. those patients who were not long-term in 1994, has already started to accumulate at a similar rate to previous cohorts (Fig. 12.3).

If we use alternative definitions of long-term patients, i.e. 'those with periods between two contacts never longer than 60 days, or 30 or 15 days', we can see that all these categories of frequent users of mental health services are accumulating over the years (Fig. 12.4). On the 1995 census day there were 164, 81 and 49 South-Verona patients who were in continuous care for one year or more, having a contact at least every two months or one month or two weeks respectively.

The South-Verona CMHS is now taking care of most psychiatric patients who, before the reform, would have been admitted to the mental hospital and become long-stay. They receive intensive and continuous community-based care (out-patient care, home visits and crisis intervention, day care) and have spells of admission to hospital (the psychiatric ward of the general hospital or the private psychiatric hospitals) when necessary. In all settings but the private hospitals they remain under the care of the same team.

Monitoring service utilisation over the years and comparing South-Verona area with other areas with different systems of mental health care. The South-Verona PCR has been used in several studies conducted so far to

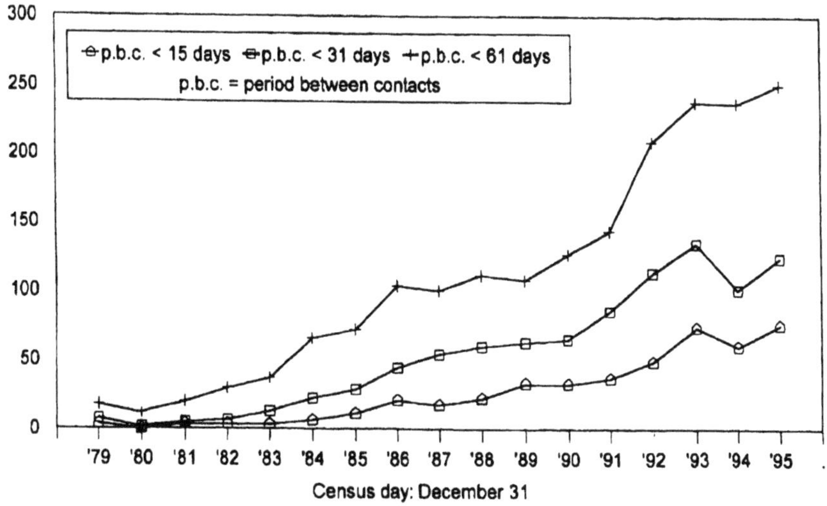

FIG. 12.4. Long-term patients with frequent contacts with psychiatric services (ratios per 1,000 adult South-Verona residents).

monitor service utilisation and patterns of care. (Tansella & Ruggeri, 1996) It has been shown that patients with a diagnosis of psychosis are more likely than other patients to be both higher users (those who have many contacts in a defined period of time) and long-term users. Service utilisation measures for the period 1983–89 were used to identify associations with socio-demographic variables from the 1981 census. The most strongly associated predictor variables, both for schizophrenia and all diagnoses were: living alone, unemployment, percentage of the total population who is dependent, and percentage divorced, separated or widowed.

Patterns of care in South-Verona have been compared with those in four other areas in Italy, in Aarhus, Denmark, Groningen, The Netherlands, and Manchester, England.

A case register study was recently completed to address the question of whether the delivery of continuity of care is different in a community-based system of care (South-Verona, Italy) as compared with a hospital-based system (Groningen, Holland). The continuity of care was measured by means of two indicators: readiness of aftercare (the time from discharge from hospital to the first day- or outpatient contact) and flexibility of care (the combination of in-, day- and outpatient care during a two-year follow-up). Both indicators showed a higher continuity of care in South-Verona (Sytema, Micciolo, & Tansella, 1997).

THE OUTCOME PROJECT

In the last few years we developed an integrated model for assessing the outcome of care routinely: the South-Verona Outcome Project. In this model, variables belonging to four main dimensions are considered: clinical variables, social variables, variables concerning the interaction with services (specifically, needs for care, satisfaction with services, family burden) and data on service utilisation and costs. Both quantitative and qualitative measures are used and the assessment for the latter is multi-axial, i.e. takes into account the perspectives of patients, relatives and professionals.

Standardised assessments take place twice a year: from April to June (wave A) and from October to December (wave B). During these periods both first-ever patients and patients already in contact with the service are assessed at the first or, at latest, second time they are seen. In wave A the assessment includes the Global Assessment of Functioning Scale (GAF), the Brief Psychiatric Rating Scale (BPRS, 'expanded version'), eight items from the Disability Assessment Scale (DAS-II) and the Camberwell Assessment of Needs (CAN). In wave B the assessment includes again GAF, BPRS, and DAS and the Lancashire Quality of Life Profile (LQL) and the Verona Service Satisfaction Scale (VSSS). Quantitative data on socio-demographic characteristics, psychiatric history and service utilisation are routinely recorded in the South-Verona PCR.

These data indicate that in South-Verona the diagnosis of psychosis is not necessarily a marker for unfavourable life circumstances and that the South-Verona CPS meets the demands of psychotic patients. Moreover, they indicate that the perspective of patients and professionals convey complementary points of view (Biggeri, Rucci, Ruggeri, & Tansella, 1996).

STUDIES FOR EVALUATING COSTS

All patients (*n*=706) who in 1992 had at least one contact with services reporting to the South-Verona psychiatric case register and received an ICD–10 diagnosis were included in a study to evaluate direct costs of care. The costs of specialist psychiatric care provided in the 365 days following the first 1992 contact were calculated using a unit cost list. For each patient, costs were calculated using dedicated software, linked to the case register and designed by our research team and were grouped by in-patient costs, sheltered accommodation costs, day-care costs, out-patient costs, and community costs. The results can be summarised as follows (Amaddeo, Beecham, Bonizzato, Fenyo, Knapp, & Tansella, 1997a; Amaddeo, Bonizzato, & Tansella, 1997b):

1. All costs, grouped by service type, were found to be significantly different ($P < 0.01$) between diagnostic groups.
2. The multivariate analyses showed that costs are significantly higher for people with a diagnosis of schizophrenia and related disorders than for people belonging to the other diagnostic groups. However, only 6% of the variation could be explained by diagnostic group alone. On the other hand, between 37 and 53% of the costs of mental health care was predicted by patients' personal characteristics and other measures recorded on the case register.

One of the main variables accounting for differences in costs between patients is previous psychiatric history, patients with longer or chronic history having higher costs. In areas where a shift has taken place from a hospital-based to a community-based system of psychiatric care it is interesting to evaluate costs of new patients, i.e. patients having their first life time psychiatric contact, for at least two reasons: First, the costs of this subgroup of patients is not subjected to interference from previous encounters with psychiatric services, including those in the old hospital-based system; lower between-patient variability and higher predictive values of cost equations can therefore be expected. Second, these patients have patterns of care that are different from those of other patients, i.e. patients already known to the services, especially the most chronic. To our knowledge no studies so far have analysed the costs of patients at the first psychiatric contact in their life (first-ever patients).

Direct costs of care provided in the 365 days following the index contact were assessed for all first-ever patients (n=299) and (for comparison) for all longer-term patients (n=768) who had at least one contact with psychiatric services over a two-year period (from January 1992 to December 1993). The results can be summarised as follows:

1. First-ever patients, in the first year after the index contact, are significantly less costly as compared with all other patients in contact with the same services during an equivalent period of time. The cost difference is confirmed for all diagnostic groups taken into account in our research. When total costs are disaggregated into their components, by type of treatment, the difference is no longer significant for in-patient care of patients with a diagnosis of schizophrenia and for out-patient care in all four diagnostic groups.
2. Known patients, as compared to first-ever, required, in all diagnostic groups, a similar amount of out-patient care, but more (and more expensive) day care and community care, which includes home visits by psychiatrists, as well as by nurses and social workers. These data

confirm that, for patients with a previous psychiatric history, all components of a community-based system of care are important, but the key component is not out-patient care, but domiciliary visits, day-care and rehabilitation programmes. The implication of these results for service organisation is that resources should be dedicated to ensure the provision of the above mentioned types of care, together with care provided by traditional out-patients departments.

3. Our data also confirm that, when analysing costs of care provided by specialist public services, there is a decreasing trend of costs from patients with diagnosis of schizophrenia and related disorders (the most expensive) to those with affective disorders and with other diagnosis. The least expensive are those with neurotic and somatoform disorders, probably because they also receive care from private psychiatrists and psychologists who do not report to the case register.
4. Between 20% and 69% of the observed inter-patient cost variation is explained statistically by individual characteristics included in cost functions. The lowest percentage of the variance explained was found in the diagnostic group "other diagnosis". On the other hand, the variance explained by individual characteristics, in more homogeneous groups, such as the group of patients with schizophrenia and related disorders, is much higher (69%).
5. Analysing the costs of all patients with a diagnosis of schizophrenia and related disorders who had at least one contact in the two year period 1992–1993, we found that for more than 90% of patients the costs are lower than those of continuous one year stay in a state mental hospital (*manicomio*). For 3.6% the costs are higher than those for a continuous one year stay in a *manicomio* and lower than those for one year stay in a private psychiatric clinic. For 3.1% the costs are higher than those for a one year stay in a private clinic and lower than those for a one year stay in a psychiatric ward of a general hospital. Finally, for 3% of patients the costs are higher than those of one year of continuous care in the most expensive in-patient institution.
6. Patients with a longer psychiatric history cost significantly more than shorter-term patients.

Two limitations of the studies reported above have to be underlined. First, being case register studies, only costs of care as provided by the specialist psychiatric system, i.e. by services and agencies reporting to the case register, not the total societal costs are assessed. Second, the cost evaluation was limited to the first year following the index contact; no information was provided on costs of psychiatric care over longer periods. While it would be easy to solve the second problem, using the present methodology in this or in a similar cohort of first-ever patients followed for a longer period of time, the first limitation can be unravelled only by using appropriate instruments such as the Client Service Receipt Interview (CSRI) and a prospective research design. Both types of research are actually in progress in Verona.

FUTURE CHALLENGES

New problems are likely to enter the picture in the next few years, in particular those related to social changes and consequent instability. So far, in Verona, as well as in the rest of the country, with the possible exception of large cities, and of (relatively small) areas massively infiltrated by the refugees coming from former Yugoslavia, Albania, and eastern Europe in general, the structure of society has providentially remained steady.

The family, including the extended one, has continued to be a solid institution all over the country, thus both limiting the magnitude of problems commonly found in broken families, and providing an invaluable resource of accommodation and support for the mentally ill. However, such favourable conditions are not taken for granted even in the short run, and mental health services are likely to have to respond to ever-growing family-related distress, and to provide for the people with mental disorders abandoned by families.

Mental health services will also have to prepare for a growing number of disadvantaged people, like the old, the immigrants, and the poor. A common question asked by foreign professionals visiting our service is related to the care, especially residential care, of the elderly. Our answer is that we are lucky for the social reasons seen above, but that we are aware it will not be like that for ever! And the number of the old is rapidly increasing: the current political turmoil around the reform of the seniority-pension system is just one aspect of the broader, dramatic problems of an ageing society.

Immigration from Maghreb, western Africa, and especially eastern Europe, is rapidly changing the shape of our society. The Italian, who has been dormant for centuries, far from racial issues, and idling over semi-serious prejudices between the north and the south, is now rapidly discovering the amenities of a multi-racial society. Minority-specific mental health problems are still of modest scale, probably because the fittest individuals have succeeded to immigrate, but services have to prepare to face a completely new set of demands.

Cutting costs will be a painful must for mental health services in the coming years. Between 1991 and 1993 a number of laws remodelled the National Health Service: each ULSS has been reorganised as an enterprise, a business organisation, with strict budgetary constraints. All medium-to-large scale hospitals have become enterprises themselves, independent of the ULSS where they are located.

These changes may create difficulties for mental health services. An unprecedented concern for containing expenses, typical of the new ULSS enterprises, will put mental health at a disadvantage with regard to other more lucrative and politically attractive medical specialities. In addition, where the hospital has become independent of the ULSS, mental health care is usually provided by separate in-patient and community services, with understandable risks for the continuity of care. Our Service has succeeded in remaining one, but has to face administrative divisions of responsibility and a shrinking budget anyway.

We foresee that the service will become more and more structured and efficiency oriented. The increasing number of workers and programmes involved demand more coordination and more structure. We expect that continuity of care will depend more on collaboration between workers and programmes rather than on the same worker performing different roles and remaining the sole link for the user. Specialisation and cooperation will progressively replace an up-to-now prevalent generalist approach.

At the same time, there will likely be an increasing user participation and responsibility in the service. The user self-help group is already conjointly operating with the service. Whether it will become more attached or more independent remains to be seen. In any case users (and families) will ask for more say in programming and evaluating facilities, and interventions. User participation in the decision process is still a question of personal relationships and good will, rather than an acknowledged and established rule in the Italian health (including mental health) system. Our service may become a model in this respect by simply capitalising on existing resources, including the user self-help association.

In conclusion, we may expect more challenges, especially in social and economic terms, and have to be ready to optimise existing resources: they are not going to increase, and may possibly decrease. However, the solid and comprehensive structure of the service, and its long-lasting experience, have the numbers to face such future challenges.

CONCLUSIONS

It is often stated that it is now necessary for health services, including services for the mentally ill, to provide accurate, routinely collected data on the clinical activities carried out and their outcome, in order to evaluate them. It is also widely recognised that these data, to be compared with those from other areas, should be epidemiologically based. To conclude this chapter we should stress that both monitoring and evaluating mental health services using an epidemiological approach require extra financial resources and availability of scientific competence and skills. Therefore, before embarking on such a programme, its costs and the practicability of implementing and running it should be carefully evaluated. The advantages of this policy are clear: it may assist the administrators in deciding what services are cost-effective (which should not be interpreted as cost-saving) and it makes it possible for mental health professionals to ensure that the evidence-based foundation for planning and evaluating mental health services is counter-balanced by ethically-based clinical values; these values, as for example accountability, accessibility, coordination, continuity of care, should be made explicit and confirmed by the general organisation of the service as well as by monitored daily service activities (Tansella & Thornicroft, 1998).

ACKNOWLEDGEMENTS

We are grateful to our many colleagues in the Institute of Psychiatry of the University of Verona as well as in many other scientific institutions in Italy and abroad who helped us in collecting data and in the analyses and collaborated in the evaluative studies conducted in the last 18 years in South-Verona. They are too many and it is impossible to mention them all.

The main evaluative studies reported here have been funded by the *Ministero dell'Universita e della Ricerca Scientifica, Roma*, by the *Consiglio Nazionale delle Ricerche (CNR), Roma* and by the *Assessorato alla Sanita, Regione Veneto, Venezia*. The preparation of this chapter was supported by the *Fondazione Cassa di Risparmio di Verona Vicenza Belluno e Ancona, Progetto Sanita* 1996–1997, Grant 'The role of social factors on onset, course and outcome of mental disorders: An epidemiological approach' to Professor Michele Tansella.

REFERENCES

Amaddeo, F., Beecham, J., Bonizzato, P., Fenyo, A., Knapp, M.J.R., & Tansella, M. (1997a). The use of a case register for evaluating the costs of psychiatric care. *Acta Psychiatrica Scandinavica, 95*, 189–198.

Amaddeo, F., Beecham, J., Bonizzato, P., Fenyo, A., Tansella, M., & Knapp, M. (1998). The cost of community-based psychiatric care for first-ever patients: A case-register study. *Psychological Medicine, 28*, 173–183.

Amaddeo, F., Bonizzato, P., & Tansella, M. (1997b). Psychiatric case registers for monitoring service utilisation and evaluating its costs. In M.Tansella (Ed.) *Making Rational Mental Health Services* (pp. 177–198). Roma: Il Pensiero Scientifico Editore.

Biggeri, A., Rucci, P., Ruggeri, M., & Tansella, M. (1996). Multidimensional assessment of outcome. The analysis of conditional independence as an integrated statistical tool to model the relationships between variables. In G. Thornicroft & M. Tansella (Eds) *Mental Health Outcome Measures* (pp. 207–216). Heidelberg: Springer-Verlag.

Comune di Verona (1996). *Annuario Statistico 1995.* Comune di Verona, Verona: Ufficio di Statistica.

ISTAT (1994). *Popolazione e Abitazioni. Fascicolo Provinciale Verona, 13° Censimento Generale della Popolazione e delle Abitazioni.* Roma: Istituto Nazionale di Statistica.

ISTAT (1995). *Popolazione e Abitazioni. Fascicolo Nazionale Italia, 13° Censimento Generale della Popolazione e delle Abitazioni.* Roma: Istituto Nazionale di Statistica.

ISTAT (1996). *Italian Statistical Abstract, 1994.* Roma: Istituto Nazionale di Statistica.

Sytema, S., Micciolo, R., & Tansella, M. (1997). Continuity of care for patients with schizophrenia and related disorders: a comparative South-Verona and Groningen case-register study. *Psychological Medicine, 27,* 1355–1362.

Tansella, M. (Ed.) (1991). *Community-based psychiatry: Long-term patterns of care in South-Verona. Psychological Medicine Monograph Supplement 19.* Cambridge: Cambridge University Press.

Tansella, M. (1993). The Research Unit of the Servizio di Psicologia Medica at the Institute of the University of Verona, 1980–1991. *Psychological Medicine, 23,* 239–247.

Tansella, M. & Ruggeri, M. (1996). Monitoring and evaluating a community-based service. In R. Smith & M. Peckham (Eds), *The Scientific Basis of Health Services* (pp. 160–169). London: British Medical Journal.

Tansella, M. & Thornicroft, G. (1998). A conceptual framework for mental health services: the matrix model. *Psychological Medicine, 28,* 503–508.

Tansella, M. & Williams, P. (1989). The spectrum of psychiatric morbidity in a defined geographical area. *Psychological Medicine, 19,* 765–770.

Tansella, M. & Zimmermann Tansella, Ch. (1988). From mental hospitals to alternative community services. In J.C. Howells (Ed.), *Modern perspectives in clinical psychiatry.* (pp. 130–148). New York: Brunner Mazel.

Thornicroft, G. & Tansella, M. (in press). *The mental health matrix. A pragmatic guide to improve services.* Cambridge: Cambridge University Press.

CHAPTER THIRTEEN

Messages from the workshops

David Goldberg and Graham Thornicroft
Institute of Psychiatry, London, UK

There were 42 workshops offering participants to the conference a choice of 7 after each group of plenary talks. They were our principal way of creating a dialogue between users and providers of mental illness services. The topics dealt with in the workshops had been decided upon during a series of joint meetings between policy makers, providers and users during the three months preceding the conference. All suggestions for workshops came from the users themselves, but were then narrowed down by a wider group of users and officials from both the King's Fund and the Maudsley. The themes were both about ends like personal autonomy and self-determination, and means such as advocacy, participation, volunteering, employment and single agency working.

Each workshop kicked off with three 10-minute talks, one by a user, and two by mental health experts from London, another from elsewhere in the UK or from one of the 10 cities; and each one was chaired by a facilitator. There was a striking difference between the atmosphere on the first day of the conference, and that on the last two days. Early on, there was often a confrontational atmosphere, each side tending to fall back on well-prepared positions: a genuine dialogue was difficult in these conditions. However, confidence was soon established as it became clear that both providers and managers wished to hear what users had to say—and it was soon apparent that each side had much to learn from the other.

The users—whether or not they had been asked to prepare something—

were soon accepted as autonomous participants. By learning to work collaboratively with professionals, managers and volunteers they created a much more powerful voice in the system, and participants from the 10 cities all reinforced this view. It was stressed by users that personal autonomy was still important even when they were acutely ill; that what matters at these times is 'me, here, now' rather than the official records and procedures. The message from users is that their opinions should be taken into account when treatment is planned, and their consent should be sought if information is to be passed to others. Problems need to be resolved about the information that the user's carer has a right to know, if they are to share responsibility for the user's future health.

The contribution that can be made by volunteers was a theme that occurred repeatedly, and users were seen to be aiming at active citizenship, forming networks and alliances to help in this respect. Volunteers were seen as introducing real friendship, and using different skills—with a chance to open the emotional side of things that tends to be soft pedalled by the professionals.

Although shortage of resources was a recurrent theme, no-one dwelled upon it: the emphasis always being on what more could be achieved even with existing resources, if both professional attitudes and usual working practices could be altered. The workshop on London's Mental Health confirmed many of the themes that had already been highlighted by the King's Fund Report, including the need for an authority that could take a complete overview of London's problems; the wearing down of the divisions between health and social care, specialist and primary care, and statutory and voluntary care; the need for more creative approaches to community housing. We will highlight some recurrent themes in three particular areas.

IMPROVEMENTS TO THE COMMUNITY MENTAL HEALTH SERVICES

A 24-hour community psychiatric outreach service for the inner city not only provided care for the mentally ill homeless, but had been shown to have decreased admissions to hospital relative to a part of the city with no such service. Intensive and assertive community care in Sydney reduced hospital bed use for the 'revolving door' patients who had previously been difficult to treat and non-compliant with medication. There seemed to be clear messages for London here: and extended hours service can undertake emergency home assessment at any time, and often support and treat the mentally ill at home; they are found to be preferable to ambulance or police services, that would tend to deal with emergencies by removing the patient from the home environment. We heard from Madison, Wisconsin that 75%

of people in crisis can be diverted from seeking in-patient care, providing that there is a 24-hour crisis helpline.

Both the teams from the USA, and the team from Verona, described how non-professionals can make valuable contributions as part of the mental health teams—either by providing supportive care, or by acting as staff in community residential facilities.

THE NEED FOR HOUSING

The workshop on residential facilities stressed the range of facilities needed, and the fact that poverty and lack of choice prevent people from breaking free from the mental health system. Ethnic minority groups were seen as being especially disadvantaged by lack of choice. The lack of a proper range of suitable accommodation both delays discharge and causes relapses. We heard from users who had waited—either in hospital or homeless—for as long as 18 months for suitable accommodation in the community.

Ideal arrangements would include both individual and shared space to balance the need for privacy with opportunities for social interaction and the prevention of isolation. Three sorts of need were identified: facilities that could be available to deal with crises, the need for respite care, and the provision of asylum and shelter in a non-medical setting.

The team from Amsterdam saw clear links between inappropriate living arrangements and homelessness, and this theme was emphasised by HART, the housing assessment and rehabilitation team from Hackney, London. This team had been jointly commissioned by health and social services, but the majority of its funding comes from the Department of Health. This team works with people who have become disengaged from usually mental health services—either being rejected by them or because they wished to avoid contact with them. The first team was set up in 1994, and some teams now work with street sleepers, others work with those in hostel or temporary accommodation. There is both direct work with clients and inter-agency working. An evaluation had shown that all clients were suffering from (usually severe) mental disorders, but that about a half had alcohol or drug problems in addition. Nevertheless, it had proved possible to place 60% of referrals either in permanent housing or in another agency pending placement.

MENTAL HEALTH IN PRIMARY CARE

Several workshops touched on this important theme, and users had much to say about the importance of the quality of the first person met—most usually a general practitioner. Users were generally quite prepared to see staff other than the GP after their first interview, and there was a general appreciation that they did not want to waste the doctor's time—although they did not want to feel rushed, either. If the doctor is to handle a depressed patient, consideration should be given to a longer appointment, perhaps at the end of a surgery. Those GPs who were thought to exemplify good practice had certain common characteristics: they were sympathetic, they listened, and allowed users enough time to describe their problems, they were concerned about the patient's life-style and recent stressful life events, and they gave detailed advice about management and any medical treatment. Those GPs not living up to these high standards were thought to lack sufficient specialist knowledge about depression and its treatment, gave users poor information, and generally lacked sensitivity. Improved liaison between primary care teams and local voluntary groups was thought to broaden the choice that could be offered to users. A more active role in the administration of cost-effective forms of treatment were seen both for practice nurses, and for re-trained counsellors.

For those with more severe disorders, good liaison between primary care and the CMH teams was thought to be important, and we heard about several arrangements which were thought to improve the interface between the two services. These included using the GP's surgery address rather than the users as a basis for catchment areas, having link workers assigned to sets of GPs by the specialist mental health team, providing training to primary care team members in modern forms of effective treatment, and jointly contributing to 'good practice protocols' for the management of common disorders. Psychiatrists and psychologists were thought to need to learn to share their skills with staff in primary care, and greater investment was needed to develop an integrated system. The future availability of self-treatment by manuals, computer or CD-ROMs was also described.

USER PARTICIPATION

An important workshop on this theme saw this as ensuring a service that was focused on the needs of users, and stressed the therapeutic value of such activities: users feel that they are not merely participating with professionals, but contributing to the processes of their own recovery. Coping skills can be developed, and experiences shared. Increased participation by users was thought to shift policies and contribute to the training of the mental health professionals, as well as helping to destigmatise mental illness.

Users acknowledged the need to trust others when they were too ill, or too distressed, to manage themselves—but thought that the support of an advocate or trusted friend was crucial to this process. Advocacy was mentioned several times: it needs to remain truly independent, and to be effective, reliable, and credible. Discussing problems of staff burnout, users mentioned that they were not so trapped as most of the professionals seemed to be, as they could choose to live outside the system if they chose.

DIVERGENT THEMES

We did not succeed in agreeing about everything. Users thought that they should play an important role in deciding what constituted a cost-effective treatment; while professionals generally thought that while such studies are based upon results of outcomes with sets of individual users, that the techniques are complex, and should try to be as objective as possible. Users also thought that psychiatrists and other professionals should not be thought of as being predominantly—still less solely—responsible for the actions of users while they were ill. The current mental health services were found to consume the time, energy and goodwill of staff, and to be too medically focused. It irked many users that a psychiatrist might have the final say in depriving them of their liberty.

Psychiatrists, on the other hand, were concerned about being made to be responsible for situations in the community which their teams were unable to cope with, given the level of resource and staffing levels that are currently available to them. Much of the low morale and burnout was attributed to the culture of blame that continues to surround work with severely mentally ill users. Furthermore, it is still the consultant psychiatrist who must appear before the coroner's court or the Committee of Enquiry: until society changes its expectations, it will be necessary for final decisions about deprivation of liberty to be made by the psychiatrist who may be held ultimately responsible for the user's care.

CHAPTER FOURTEEN

Overview and emerging themes

David Goldberg and Graham Thornicroft
Institute of Psychiatry, London, UK

OVERALL COMPARISONS BETWEEN THE CITIES

We saw in Chapter 1 that cities are getting bigger: by the year 2015, it is estimated that Lagos, Bombay, Jakarta, and Sao Paulo are predicted to have populations of 24.4, 27.4, 21.2 and 20.8 million respectively (Lancet, 1996). None of the cities that came to the conference were anything like this size, and the task of organising a mental health system which is equitable and comprehensive on this scale is a formidable one. As cities get larger, they lose their human scale, and for this reason we have presented findings for smaller cities like Baltimore, Madison and Verona which have, in their different ways, planned comprehensive community mental health services.

It can be seen from Fig. 14.1 that the largest cities represented at the conference were London and Tehran, and it is perhaps no accident that neither of these cities has yet achieved a well planned, city-wide community mental health service. The largest of the cities to have come nearest to this ideal is Sydney, while one has to look at smaller cities for good examples of such services.

However, size alone provides a poor indicator of the complexity of the problems faced by the planners in each city: we have seen in Chapter 2 the extent of social deprivation and diversity of a city the size of London. In comparative terms, the area occupied by London is similar to that of

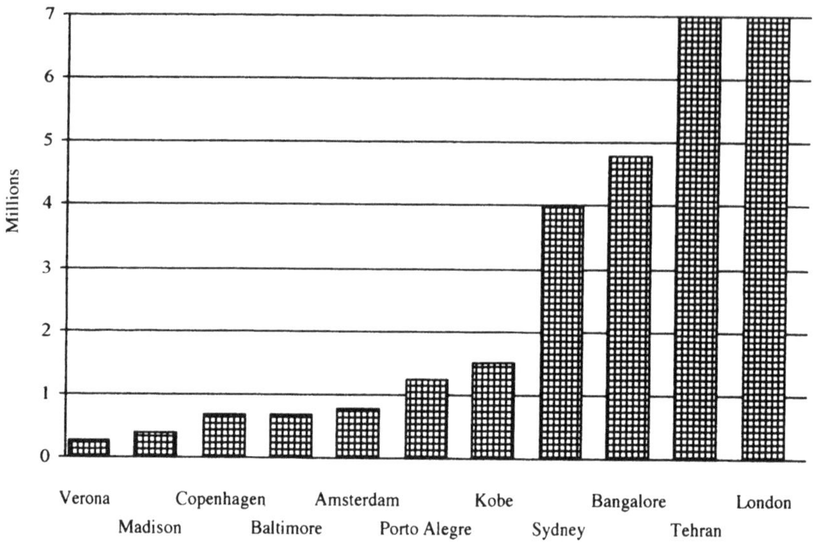

FIG. 14.1. Size of the population in the 11 cities.

Sydney—so that the density of population is that much greater in London. Indeed, Sydney lingers in the memory not only as a good place to live (in public health terms, of course!) but as a city with well staffed and well integrated community teams, who meet one another every day, and run a well thought out service.

Bangalore, Baltimore, London, and Tehran all have much higher rates of social deprivation to deal with, and this will be reflected in the load upon their services. Since social deprivation is likely to be a feature of the future megalopolis (see Chapter 1), the ways in which the problem has been dealt with so far are of great interest. Services for the whole population are poorly provided in both Bangalore and Tehran, although the latter city is clearly changing very rapidly. However, both of these are heavily reliant on primary care, and we argue that by itself this is likely to be insufficient. Baltimore appears to offer an exciting model for collaboration across the various agencies concerned with mental health services, as well as offering a model for collaboration between university departments and mental health services.

THE RESOURCES DEVOTED TO HEALTH

One index of the importance shown to health is the proportion of the gross domestic product (GDP) spent on health services. Of the paired histograms in Fig. 14.2, the left hand one for each city represents the proportion of

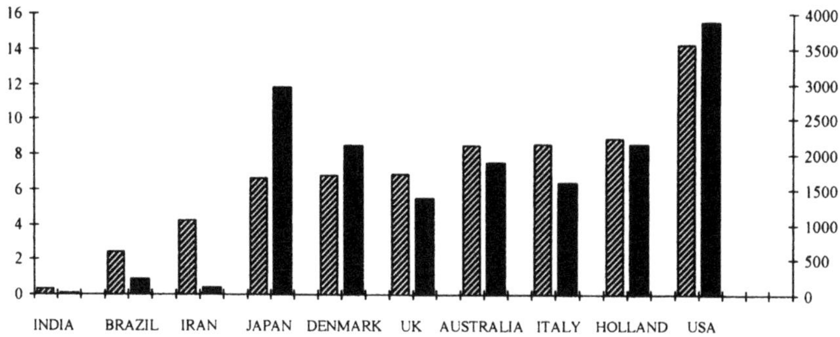

FIG. 14.2. Percentage of gross domestic product spent on health, with countries arranged in rank order with the lowest to the left, and the highest to the right, for 10 countries represented at the conference. The black histograms show the value of the health spend, per head of population, in US dollars.

gross domestic product spent on health, and are arranged in rank order, with India on the left with the lowest and USA on the right with the highest—with no less than 14.2% of its GDP spent on health. It is perhaps inevitable that in all the countries with lesser expenditure (like India, Iran, and Brazil) there has been more of a 'let's start with a clean sheet' approach to the mental illness services.

It is again no accident that the three countries whose cities come nearest to the ideal of a comprehensive community service—in Italy, the USA and Australia—all spend more than 8% of their GDP on health, and spend more on health per capita than the UK.

There are very real differences between the health care systems of the countries spending between 6 and 8% of their GDP on health, but we must remember that governments are able to allow health costs to increase, or to hold them steady, or even gradually to reduce them: but they inherit a pattern of spending from their predecessors; and this is in any case largely determined by the clinical resources available to each particular country.

The major shortcoming of these data is that there are immense variations between countries in the size of their GDP, so that a better measure, in many ways, is the spending for an average citizen during the course of a year—and this is shown on the right hand of the paired histograms. The two big spenders are USA and Japan; but they spend their money on rather different things, as we shall see. The four European countries and Australia emerge as a middle group—though it is noteworthy that the UK spends the least in this group. Of course, these data do not allow exact comparisons either, since $100 will buy much more health care in India than it does in the USA.

We also need to consider time trends in expenditure on health: these show steady rises with time in most countries for which data are available except the UK: in this country expenditure was held remarkably steady at 6.1% for some years, and has only experienced a modest increase in the past two years as an impending general election caused our previous government to relax its restrictions on health spending. Among the developed countries, the UK emerges as the only country to be controlling health expenditures with any success; and to be remarkably frugal spenders on health care in general.

Hospital beds are the biggest single item in any health budget, and in the developing world beds have been greatly reduced to achieve greater cost-effectiveness by shortening average length of stay. Figure 14.3 shows the total number of hospital beds per 100,000 at risk, once more arranged in rank order. In view of its high health spend, one might therefore have expected to find the USA at the top of this list, but it has severely restricted hospital beds in an attempt to control escalating health expenditure. Japan, Holland and Australia have the most beds, while Iran and India have the fewest. Bed numbers are still rising in Japan, and this is probably related to the high value of the health spend per head of population, shown in Fig. 14.2, along with the financial incentives offered to the owners of private psychiatric hospitals.

However, it is psychiatric beds that are of particular interest, and here the local trends are somewhat different. The extent to which the old mental hospitals have been replaced is a powerful determinant of total mental health service costs, as many governments have already discovered. It is not possible to present comparative data on the exact size of the mental health spend in each city, as this information is not generally available.

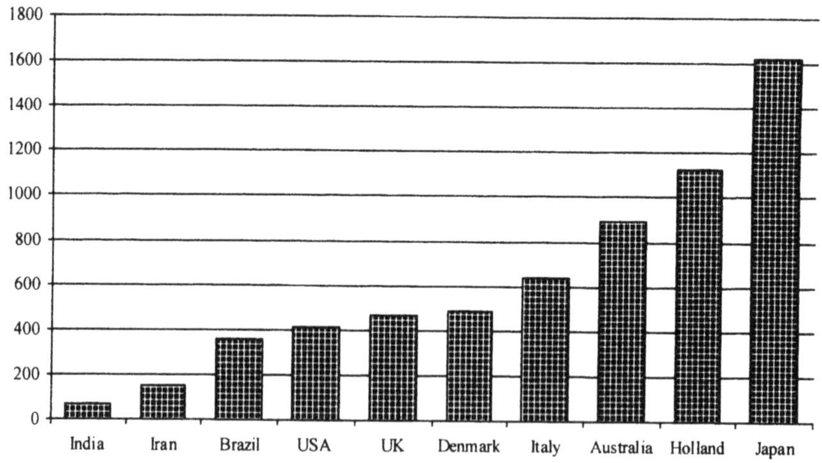

FIG. 14.3. Total hospital beds per 100,000 at risk: 10 countries in ascending rank order.

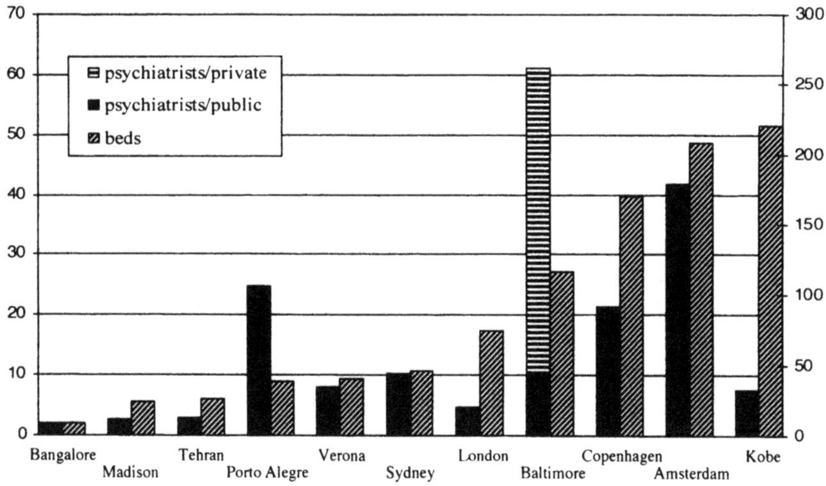

FIG. 14.4. The right hand histograms show psychiatric beds per 100,000 population, arranged in ascending rank order. The histograms on the left show numbers of psychiatrists available in each city; although data for Madison only relate to the public sector services.

We might have supposed that psychiatric beds would be in some fairly predictable proportion to total health service beds: but different countries have made very different progress in closing down their mental hospitals. Kobe has the greatest number of beds, and their numbers continue to increase. Amsterdam and Copenhagen also have relatively high rates, despite the progress described in earlier chapters. As we have heard, the two latter European countries have on the whole been more cautious about changing their mental health delivery systems. The main difference between Amsterdam and Kobe is that Amsterdam is closing its beds, while those in Japan are still booming.

Sydney, we note, is not alone in having made do with few beds, it is actually in quite good company. Sydney, Verona and Porto Alegre have each adopted radical revisions of their mental health systems, and are making do with far fewer beds than in inner London, but rather more than outer London. On the other hand, the social correlates of mental ill-health are very much less severe in these cities than they are in inner London.

The two American cities appear very different: but once more, Baltimore resembles London in having high indices of social disadvantage, and large ethnic minority populations, in contrast to Madison. Nonetheless, Madison's 24 beds will be looked at with envy from Verona: both are pleasant, smallish cities surrounded by attractive countryside, and with relatively low levels of social deprivation. However, the Madison figures do not include private beds, which do exist in the city.

Numbers of psychiatrists per 100,000 at risk are also widely variable. Ideally, one should consider whole time equivalents rather than people—but such data are only available in two of the cities: so these data relate to overall numbers of people, trainees excluded. Psychiatrists appear amazingly plentiful—by British standards, at any rate—in Baltimore, Kobe, Amsterdam and Copenhagen: but psychiatrists working in the public sector are no more common in Baltimore than in London or Sydney. The relatively high numbers in Amsterdam may reflect the independence of the RIAGGS and the hospital system. Porto Alegre and Copenhagen have numbers well above average; while low numbers are seen in London and the developing countries.

It is worth noticing that there is no relationship between numbers of psychiatrists and numbers of psychiatric beds: a relatively well-resourced, mental health orientated population of a city like Baltimore can support large numbers of psychiatrists despite having restricted its beds, while in Kobe a relatively small number of psychiatrists are using a large number of beds.

It is difficult to make comparisons about other mental health staff, as figures are not generally available. However, compared with other cities who have provided data, Croydon in London appears to be relatively short of professional staff to run its service (the figures for Porto Alegre and Madison are incomplete, and thus cannot be compared directly).

It can be seen from Table 14.1 that London has far fewer nurses than Copenhagen (where no distinction is made between ward and community nurses), and fewer community nurses than Verona. The overall numbers of

TABLE 14.1
Table Showing Staff Available per 100,000 Population at Risk in Three Cities

Staff type	*Copenhagen*	*London (Croydon)*	*Verona*
Psychiatrists:			
Whole time equivalents	–	4.1	7.93
Different individuals	30	–	11.00
Psychologists	9	0.93	4.43
Ward nurses	100	39.0	19.24
Community nurses	–	8.6	17.66
Occupational therapists	10	3.6	–
Social workers	10	5.0	2.44
Mental health Aides	–	–	16.50
Others	66	–	1.83
Total	225	62.3	73.1

staff are also less in London than either of the other cities. These figures reflect the problems in delivering effective community care in London, referred to in Chapter 2.

MESSAGES FOR LONDON

In London, the dismemberment of the Greater London Council (a London-wide local government authority) has meant that social services offered to Londoners vary widely between different boroughs, and the division of the city into North and South divisions of the NHS Executive, with many different purchasing authorities, has meant that mental health services are also very heterogeneous—as we described in Chapter 2. The arrival of a single London office of government, promised by our new Labour government, taken together with a determination for health authorities to work closely with local authority social services and housing departments, and the criminal justice system in planning services, may yet cause substantial improvements in community mental health services (Department of Health, 1998).

By contrast with the other cities, London is very heterogeneous, with large areas of highly socially deprived population, high use of illicit drugs, high unemployment, and large refugee and ethnic minority populations. It attempts to provide services with a relatively low mental health spend, and without large numbers of psychiatrists or other professional staff. In contrast with other developed countries, the services in London are under-resourced, and are short of both staff and living accommodation for users in the community. All who work in its mental health services, and all those who use the services, or whose family uses them, must fervently hope that more resource is made available by mental health purchasers, using the additional resource soon to be made available to socially deprived areas by our new government.

In the meantime, we must study the strong points of other services, to see which might be incorporated in our own services; and those from other cities must also look for examples of good practice from each other.

USE OF NON-PROFESSIONAL STAFF

With low morale among staff, with progressive shortages of ALL mental health professions in deprived city areas, the findings reported from Baltimore and Verona on the use of non-professional staff will be read with great interest in the UK. Six of the cities are already using such staff, and many of the contributions they can make are extremely valuable. It is up to each service to ask itself what can be achieved without the use of highly trained staff—so that they can be used for those functions that need to be carried out by professionals.

HOUSING IN THE COMMUNITY

Most of the cities with developed services have described such services, but those in the USA stand out, as examples of what can be achieved by strong central purchasers, able to purchase both health and social care from the same budget. The sheer scale of what has been done in these cities is of great interest elsewhere. Crisis residential alternatives to admission in Baltimore is an especially interesting development, which can be found in the Baltimore chapter.

In terms of the provision of unsupported accommodation for people suffering from mental illnesses, it has long been recognised that such people often also suffer from profound reductions in their material standard of living, and that this is associated in less regulated societies with a progressive 'zoning' of their places of residence. In other words, people who are most disabled by mental illnesses can only afford to live in the poorest types of accommodation, so that ghetto-isation occurs. In a sense, this is a form of social exclusion: formerly patients were confined to impoverished and separate institutions—'marginalisation within the asylum'; whereas more recently such patients are likely to be confined to impoverished areas which they share with others who do not have the economic means to afford anything better—'marginalisation within the community'.

Dear and Wolch (1987) see close parallels in these two types of marginalisation. They argue that professional care for the sick and needy has always proceeded from fundamental principles of isolation and geographical separation of such individuals. In their view, such isolation has four principal hallmarks: enclosure, partitioning, identification of functioning sites, and ranking. The operation of such market forces, combined with public opposition to new mental health facilities can find expression through local government planning procedures which address the question of where to locate new services. A frequent response to this question is one of conflict avoidance by seeking uncontested sites, with the consequent concentration of patients and other marginalised groups in to 'zones of dependence', which Dear and Wolch call 'service-dependent population ghettos'. This tendency is one of exclusion from the mainstream of social opportunities and so runs directly counter to one of the central themes of this book: that patients with (especially severe) mental illness should not be marginalised and excluded from, but be welcomed and included within the challenges and richness of normal social life.

The ways in which such social forces (including most importantly the placements policies of local government housing departments) combine to effect where people with mental health problems live are poorly researched (Elliot, Cuzick, English & Stern, 1992). What is clear however, is that they offer one manifestation, in this case spatial, which indicates the low value attached in most economically developed countries to the mentally ill (Harvey, 1996).

PERFORMANCE INDICATORS IN MADISON

Of particular interest are some of the performance indicators used in Madison. What British purchaser could expect that 80% of the budget was to be spent in the community? But then, which British purchasers are able to control the residential and other services made available by local authorities? Those in other cities who say 'this isn't how things are done in my city' perhaps should ask themselves 'why not?'. It is likely that only a merged health, housing and social services budget for the mentally ill, will allow a serious shift of resource into facilities in the community.

CONTRIBUTIONS BY USERS

Of enormous importance to us here are the contributions that can be made by users themselves. 'Reciprocal supported accommodation', where one user temporarily takes in another going through a crisis; consumer advocates, and 'On Our Own in Baltimore', the active involvement of users in the services at Porto Alegre and Amsterdam, the 'Consumer Councils' of Copenhagen and the 'Hermit Crabs' of Kobe, are all exciting examples of this. We also heard of the employment of users as direct service providers, and having users on staff selection panels.

PSYCHIATRY LIMITED

A chill note was sounded by Gavin Andrews, when he remarks in his chapter on Sydney that psychiatric services are not a resource for bad behaviour. The same idea is taken up in other cities as well: in Copenhagen, Marianne Kastrup tells us that the non-psychotic are only helped 'to the extent that there is surplus capacity'; and we have seen that the fascinating service in Baltimore is supplemented to a degree probably only ever found in the USA by a huge number of private psychiatrists. These trends are not pointed out from a position of superiority, as London is going the same way—and it isn't clear whether anyone cares. Community mental health services in Britain are becoming focused on the dangerous and the disruptive, while the wider service is starved of resource: since the prioritised patients *have* to be treated. However, such patients are a tiny minority of those who can benefit from good mental health care; and this message should be heard loud and clear; as otherwise we shall drift into a kind of service that no-one really wants, staffed by a generation of new 'alienists'.

INTERESTING INNOVATIONS

There are some interesting developments in particular cities that do not seem to be all that common in other places. 'Task groups' for difficult patients, and the use of group homes to provide day-care in Verona; the use of rating scales by front line staff in their routine work in Baltimore; the self-help groups for families of people with schizophrenia in Bangalore; and the demonstration that in New South Wales the least well resourced service appeared to be the most cost effective—will all excite considerable attention.

Patients with both psychotic symptoms and drug abuse ('dual diagnosis' patients) pose a severe challenge to any community mental health service. Once more, the two American cities seem especially interesting here, with special services for these patients, with apparently good results.

LEVELS OF SEVERITY *VS* GEOGRAPHIC CATCHMENT AREAS

A lively point of difference between the cities is concerned with those cities—like Baltimore and Madison—that stratify their services by the level of intensity of service that patients require, as opposed to those—like Verona and Copenhagen—that arrange their services entirely by geographic catchment areas. It is noteworthy that both the north American services have gone furthest in inter-agency collaboration, and have centralised mental health administrative arrangements, capable of purchasing services from a wide variety of providers.

London is unlike either of these, as it usually has a number of specialist services—such as services for children, for the elderly, for those with forensic problems, and for drug and alcohol dependence—in addition to a community oriented service for adult mental illness. It is not clear that further subdividing the latter service by degree of dependence of the patient would offer any real benefits to Londoners.

PRIMARY CARE

We saw from Chapter 1 that it is no longer sufficient to model total health needs solely on primary care service. It is worth rehearsing the reasons why this must be so. Although the bulk of common disorders have to be treated in primary care, the range of skills needed for a comprehensive treatment services are not to be found there—as these include complex psychotherapies, administration of novel anti-psychotic and mood stabilising medications, and the humane management of suicidal, homicidal, and violently disturbed psychotic patients. Assessment procedures not available in primary care include neuro-psychological and neuro-psychiatric assessment, brain imaging, rehabilitation, and day hospital facilities. Nor is the necessary expertise in dealing with patients with mental disorders sufficiently widely distributed in primary care: although some practices offer excellent facilities, many others fall far short of the necessary standards.

Gavin Andrews wonders whether money is being spent on the right things. If his arguments found favour with his government, maybe soon Australian health dollars will be removed from that excellent mental health service he describes in his chapter, and be put into primary care for the treatment of anxious depression.

While there is a great deal to be said in favour of improving the mental health skills of staff in primary care, it will always be more cost effective to provide highly specialised services required by a small proportion of the population from a well planned mental illness service. We have seen from earlier chapters that such a service requires collaboration between health, social services and local housing departments; between the public and the private sector; and between statutory and voluntary organisations. It appears that the kinds of independent mental health authorities described in Baltimore and Madison achieve this—but other systems are possible; and the arrangements in both Sydney and Verona offer possible alternatives. However—primary care is not directly involved in any of these services.

In England, and in many other countries, primary care is seen as a vital part of the mental health services, but enthusiasm for primary care must not be allowed to cause the mental health services to be neglected. What is required is that working relationships between the two services should be improved, and that each service should work closely together. There are several ways in which this could be achieved. At present, a person's street address determines the mental health service responsible for a patient's care—and this means that a GP working near the edge of two or more catchment areas may have patients looked after by several different services. This could be solved by using the GP's address, rather than the street address, as the determinant of the responsible service. This would ensure that any particular GP only had to relate to a single mental illness service.

Another relatively simple way of improving liaison is to have shared care plans, agreed between the two services for each patient with a long-term mental illness which may relapse in the future. The shared care plan gives details of current and alternative treatments; is explicit about who is responsible for prescribing; gives advice on what to do in an emergency; and gives full details of names and contact numbers on all staff involved in the patient's care.

A more ambitious plan (Goldberg & Gournay, 1997) is to have a 'link-worker' who is a member of the mental health team, but cares for all the patients with severe mental illness looked after by a particular doctor. The link worker provided ready access to other members of the team, and acts as a 'culture carrier' for providing details of training courses in mental health skills to interested members of the primary care team.

In London, it is likely that mental health services will become progressively more focused on the needs of primary care, and it is possible that a shift in resource will come to us before Australia. The excellent system described in the Verona chapter seems less likely in London, as it is relatively labour intensive, and does not allow GPs to control the resource. An independent, high quality mental health system, available to respond to GPs needs—like the RIAGG system in Holland—while guaranteeing a high standard of professionalism to patients needing special treatments, seem unlikely to be adopted in England for the same reason.

CONCLUDING COMMENTS

We live in a time when advances in both public health and health technologies are ensuring that the populations of the world live longer, and require more expensive treatments. As the pattern of health expenditure changes, it is inevitable that governments will seek to produce the most cost-effective patterns of mental health expenditure. This cannot be achieved by carrying out all planning from within the health budget, and we have seen from services described in Madison and Baltimore what can be achieved by bringing all mental illness purchasing together with a single purchaser, able to commission services from health providers, from housing departments, or from social service and voluntary agencies.

The views of service users, and their carers, need to be heard when new services, or new patterns of services are planned. Only in this way will the future cities of the world inherit services which are comprehensive, and provide adequate care for the ever growing populations of our future cities.

REFERENCES

Dear, M. & Wolch, L. (1987). *Landscapes of despair.* Cambridge: Polity.

Department of Health (1998). *The future of London's Health Services.* London: HMSO.

Elliot, T.P., Cuzick, J., English, D., & Stern, R. (1992). *Geographical and environmental epidemiology. Methods for small-area Analysis.* Oxford: Oxford University Press.

Goldberg, D.P. & Gournay, K. (1997). *The psychiatrist, the general practitioner, and the burden of mental health care.* Maudsley Discussion Paper No.1. London: Institute of Psychiatry.
Harvey, D. (1996). *Justice, nature and the geography of difference.* Oxford: Blackwell.
Lancet Editorial (1996). Big cities, small targets. *Lancet, 347*, 1637.

Author index

Subject index

For Product Safety Concerns and Information please contact our EU representative GPSR@taylorandfrancis.com
Taylor & Francis Verlag GmbH, Kaufingerstraße 24, 80331 München, Germany

www.ingramcontent.com/pod-product-compliance
Ingram Content Group UK Ltd.
Pitfield, Milton Keynes, MK11 3LW, UK
UKHW020016200926
475702UK00014B/1910
9781138884496